Global Mental Health

Editors

PARAMJIT T. JOSHI
LISA M. CULLINS

CHILD AND ADOLESCENT PSYCHIATRIC CLINICS OF NORTH AMERICA

www.childpsych.theclinics.com

Consulting Editor
HARSH K. TRIVEDI

October 2015 • Volume 24 • Number 4

ELSEVIER

1600 John F. Kennedy Boulevard • Suite 1800 • Philadelphia, Pennsylvania, 19103-2899

http://www.theclinics.com

CHILD AND ADOLESCENT PSYCHIATRIC CLINICS OF NORTH AMERICA Volume 24, Number 4
October 2015 ISSN 1056–4993, ISBN-13: 978-0-323-40076-3

Editor: Lauren Boyle
Developmental Editor: Kristen Helm

Child and Adolescent Psychiatric Clinics of North America (ISSN 1056-4993) is published quarterly by Elsevier Inc., 360 Park Avenue South, New York, NY 10010-1710. Months of issue are January, April, July, and October. Business and Editorial Offices: 1600 John F. Kennedy Boulevard, Suite 1800, Philadelphia, PA 19103-2899. Periodicals postage paid at New York, NY and additional mailing offices. Subscription prices are $310.00 per year (US individuals), $491.00 per year (US institutions), $155.00 per year (US students), $360.00 per year (Canadian individuals), $598.00 per year (Canadian institutions), $200.00 per year (Canadian students), $430.00 per year (international individuals), $598.00 per year (international institutions), and $200.00 per year (international students). International air speed delivery is included in all *Clinics* subscription prices. All prices are subject to change without notice. **POSTMASTER:** Send address changes to *Child and Adolescent Psychiatric Clinics of North America*, Elsevier Health Sciences Division, Subscription Customer Service, 3251 Riverport Lane, Maryland Heights, MO 63043. **Customer Service: 1-800-654-2452 (U.S. and Canada); 314-447-8871 (outside U.S. and Canada). Fax: 314-447-8029. E-mail:** JournalsCustomerService-usa@elsevier.com **(for print support) or** journalsonlinesupport-usa@elsevier.com **(for online support).**

Reprints. For copies of 100 or more of articles in this publication, please contact the Commercial Reprints Department, Elsevier Inc., 360 Park Avenue South, New York, New York 10010-1710 Tel.: 212-633-3874; Fax: 212-633-3820, E-mail: reprints@elsevier.com.

Child and Adolescent Psychiatric Clinics of North America is covered in *MEDLINE/PubMed (Index Medicus), ISI, SSCI, Research Alert, Social Search, Current Contents,* and *EMBASE/Excerpta Medica.*

Contributors

CONSULTING EDITOR

HARSH K. TRIVEDI, MD, MBA
Executive Director and Chief Medical Officer; Behavioral Health Vice Chair for Clinical Affairs; Associate Professor of Psychiatry, Vanderbilt University School of Medicine, Nashville, Tennessee

CONSULTING EDITOR EMERITUS

ANDRÉS MARTIN, MD, MPH

FOUNDING CONSULTING EDITOR

MELVIN LEWIS, MBBS, FRCPSYCH, DCH

EDITORS

PARAMJIT T. JOSHI, MD
Endowed Professor and Chair, Department of Psychiatry and Behavioral Sciences, Children's National Medical Center; Professor of Psychiatry, Behavioral Sciences, and Pediatrics, George Washington University School of Medicine, Washington, DC

LISA M. CULLINS, MD
Director, Child and Adolescent Psychiatry Fellowship Training Program; Director, Outpatient Psychiatry Clinic, Children's National Medical Center; Assistant Professor of Psychiatry, Behavioral Sciences, and Pediatrics, George Washington University School of Medicine, Washington, DC

AUTHORS

SUSHIL BERIWAL, MD
Residency Program Director; Associate Professor of Radiation Oncology, University of Pittsburgh Cancer Institute, Pittsburgh, Pennsylvania

PAMELA Y. COLLINS, MD, MPH
Director, Office for Research on Disparities and Global Mental Health, National Institute of Mental Health (NIMH), National Institutes of Health (NIH), Bethesda, Maryland

LISA M. CULLINS, MD
Director, Child and Adolescent Psychiatry Fellowship Training Program; Director, Outpatient Psychiatry Clinic, Children's National Medical Center; Assistant Professor of Psychiatry, Behavioral Sciences, and Pediatrics, George Washington University School of Medicine, Washington, DC

JOOP DE JONG, MD, PhD
Emeritus Professor of Cultural and International Psychiatry, VU University Medical Center, Amsterdam, Amsterdam Institute for Social Science Research (AISSR), University of Amsterdam, Amsterdam, The Netherlands; Department of Psychiatry, Boston University School of Medicine, Boston, Massachusetts

JOHN A. FAYYAD, MD
Associate Professor of Psychiatry, Faculty of Medicine, Department of Psychiatry and Clinical Psychology, St George Hospital, University Medical Center, Balamand University, Institute for Development, Research, Advocacy and Applied Care (IDRAAC), Beirut, Lebanon

JOAQUIN FUENTES, MD
Chief, Child and Adolescent Psychiatry, Policlínica Gipuzkoa; Research Consultant, Gautena Autism Program, Donostia-San Sebastián, Spain

ZACHARY D. HORNE, MD
Radiation Oncology Resident, University of Pittsburgh Cancer Institute, Pittsburgh, Pennsylvania

NEHA A. JOHN-HENDERSON, PhD
Postdoctoral Scholar, Department of Psychology, University of Pittsburgh, Pittsburgh, Pennsylvania

PARAMJIT T. JOSHI, MD
Endowed Professor and Chair, Department of Psychiatry and Behavioral Sciences, Children's National Medical Center; Professor of Psychiatry, Behavioral Sciences, and Pediatrics, George Washington University School of Medicine, Washington, DC

FINZA LATIF, MD
Director of Psychiatry Consultation-Liaison Service, Children's National Health System; Assistant Professor of Psychiatry and Behavioral Sciences, George Washington University School of Medicine, Washington, DC

RUPINDER K. LEGHA, MD
Dr Mario Pagenel Fellow in Global Mental Health Service Delivery, Partners in Health; Research Fellow, Program in Global Mental Health and Social Change, Department of Global Health and Social Medicine, Harvard Medical School, Boston, Massachusetts

BENNETT L. LEVENTHAL, MD
Professor, Department of Psychiatry; Deputy Director of Child and Adolescent Psychiatry and Director of Training, Child and Adolescent Psychiatry, Langley Porter Psychiatric Institute, University of California, San Francisco, California

SAVITA MALHOTRA, MD, PhD, FAMS
Professor and Head, Child and Adolescent Psychiatry Unit, Department of Psychiatry; Dean, Postgraduate Institute of Medical Education and Research (PGIMER), Chandigarh, India

AYESHA I. MIAN, MD
Chair and Associate Professor, Department of Psychiatry, The Aga Khan University Hospital, Karachi, Pakistan

GORDANA MILAVIĆ, MD, FRCPSYCH
Co-Chair of Child and Adolescent Psychiatry Section of World Psychiatric Association; Consultant Child and Adolescent Psychiatrist, National and Specialist Services, Michael Rutter Centre, Maudsley Hospital, London, United Kingdom

ANNA E. ORDÓÑEZ, MD, MAS
Deputy Director, Office of Clinical Research, National Institute of Mental Health (NIMH), National Institutes of Health (NIH), Bethesda, Maryland

SUSANTA KUMAR PADHY, MD
Assistant Professor, Department of Psychiatry, Postgraduate Institute of Medical Education and Research (PGIMER), Chandigarh, India

NORBERT SKOKAUSKAS, MD, PhD
Professor, Child and Adolescent Psychiatry, Centre for Child and Adolescents Mental Health and Child Protection, Faculty of Medicine, Norwegian University of Science and Technology (NTNU), Trondheim, Norway

MARTINE SOLAGES, MD
Assistant Professor of Psychiatry and Pediatrics, Department of Psychiatry and Behavioral Sciences, Children's National Medical Center, Washington, DC

SUZAN J. SONG, MD, MPH, PhD(c)
Clinical Associate Professor, Department of Psychiatry, George Washington University School of Medicine, Washington, DC; Department of Psychiatry and Anthropology, Amsterdam Institute for Social Science Research (AISSR), University of Amsterdam, Amsterdam, The Netherlands

JORGE C. SRABSTEIN, MD
Medical Director, Clinic for Health Problems of Bullying; Department of Psychiatry, Children's National Medical Center, Montgomery County Outpatient Regional Center, Rockville, Maryland; Clinical Associate Professor of Psychiatry, George Washington University School of Medicine, Washington, DC

JESSICA YEATERMEYER, MD, MSc
Child and Adolescent Psychiatry Fellow, Children's National Health System, George Washington University School of Medicine, Washington, DC

Contents

with psychiatric disorders receive treatment. Resources are insufficient, inequitably distributed, and inefficiently utilized; treatment and care are often neither evidence based nor of comprehensive or of high quality. Nationally, child and adolescent mental health policies and standardized training are virtually nonexistent. This article highlights the challenges faced and discusses measures to overcome them.

The Global Implications of Bullying and Other Forms of Maltreatment, in the Context of Migratory Trends and Psychiatric Resources **799**

Jorge C. Srabstein

This article identifies countries with the highest prevalence of bullying and other forms of maltreatment and examines the significance of these epidemiologic findings in the context of migration and availability of mental health resources. The relevance of higher prevalence of bullying and other forms of maltreatment in certain parts of the world has significant public health bearing not only on the nations affected by them but worldwide, because migrants carry with them the effects of victimization. The significant risk of abuse and violence affecting immigrants may be compounded by the effects of polyvictimization.

Psychological Impact of Nuclear Disasters in Children and Adolescents **811**

Finza Latif, Jessica Yeatermeyer, Zachary D. Horne, and Sushil Beriwal

Although much has been written about the psychological impact of natural disasters, the impact of nuclear disasters has not been extensively studied in children. Nuclear disasters are unique because they are man-made and represent a failure of the safety systems put in place to contain dangerous radioactive materials. This article summarizes the available literature on 3 of the biggest nuclear disasters in history. There is a need for further investigation not only of the impact on children but also of whether the consequences are a direct result of the disaster, radiation exposure, or the psychosocial disruptions resulting from the disaster.

Global Child and Adolescent Mental Health: A Culturally Informed Focus **823**

Lisa M. Cullins and Ayesha I. Mian

There is no question that there is a significant burden of mental illness in children and families across the globe. Despite heightened awareness of the significance of global mental health and its determinants on public health, there is an increased need for innovative interventions, research, resources, and efforts devoted to this area. It has been clearly established that culture, in all of its complex dimensions and dynamics, is at the heart of this labor. In order to integrate culture into global mental health advocacy and solutions, a collaborative approach with flexibility in thinking and implementation must exist.

Index **831**

CHILD AND ADOLESCENT PSYCHIATRIC CLINICS

FORTHCOMING ISSUES

January 2016
Adjudicated Youth
Louis Kraus, *Editor*

April 2016
Prevention of Mental Health Disorders: Principles and Implementation
Aradhana Bela Sood and James Hudziak, *Editors*

July 2016
Substance Use Disorders, Part I
Ray Hsiao and Leslie Walker, *Editors*

RECENT ISSUES

July 2015
Family-Based Treatment in Child and Adolescent Psychiatry
Michelle L. Rickerby and Thomas A. Roesler, *Editors*

April 2015
School Mental Health
Margaret M. Benningfield and Sharon Hoover Stephan, *Editors*

January 2015
Top Topics in Child and Adolescent Psychiatry
Harsh K. Trivedi, *Editor*

Preface

Partnering for Our World's Children

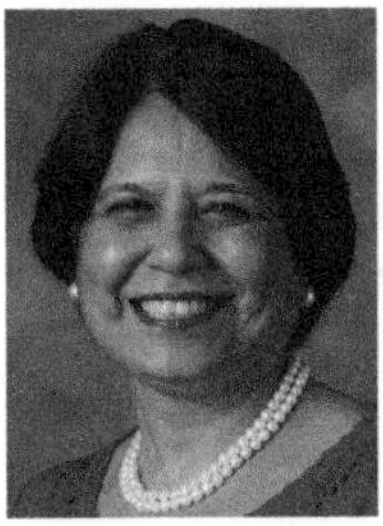
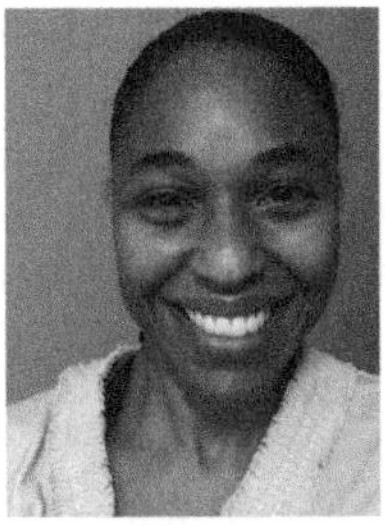

Paramjit T. Joshi, MD   Lisa M. Cullins, MD
Editors

It is a privilege for us to be the guest editors of this issue of the *Child and Adolescent Psychiatric Clinics of North America* devoted to Global Mental Health and to be among this outstanding complement of authors who have enriched this series with their contributions.

As the field of study on global mental health has evolved over the past few decades, most would agree that the mental health and well-being of all children and adolescents is a global issue. Why is it a global issue? Because no country has yet to figure out how to address the starkly unmet mental health needs of children and families on its own. The dearth of child and adolescent psychiatrists and the scarcity of resources persist worldwide. The stigma of mental health care persists worldwide. The delayed onset of treatment persists worldwide. Barriers to promote the emotional growth and well-being of all children and adolescents remain a global issue and are an undeniable crisis. So what can we do?

This issue on Global Mental Health attempts to unravel the many facets of global mental health so we can better understand the political, financial, environmental, familial, cultural, and societal underpinnings of this area of work. We believe that this collection can serve as a primer on global mental health, an introduction and overview for trainees and young clinicians, and a timely update for more seasoned clinicians. At a minimum, it will shed light on the work that still needs to be done and the progress that has been made in identifying these gaps.

The collection begins with an overview of the current status of the unmet mental health needs of our world's children and a charge that we must partner and collaborate to address them. Joshi, Leventhal, and Fuentes remind us of the past and recent atrocities that have traumatically injured our children that will have a chronic long-standing impact on their overall level of functioning in their life trajectories—requiring much needed treatment that often is not available. Furthermore, the authors shed light

Child Adolesc Psychiatric Clin N Am 24 (2015) xi–xii
http://dx.doi.org/10.1016/j.chc.2015.06.012
1056-4993/15/$ – see front matter

on burgeoning research and innovative service delivery models and powerfully impress on us that the time to act is now.

The next two articles are unique. Ordóñez and Collins leave us to contemplate the evolution of research in global mental health, the current advances, and opportunities for the future. Mian, Milavić, and Skokauskas provide both a historical and a present-day perspective on child and adolescent psychiatry training across the globe. As workforce continues to be a daunting issue as it pertains to resources and ultimately treatment, this review shares the depth and breadth of training from a global perspective.

The next six articles examine the challenges in identifying and providing psychiatric services to special populations of youth. Joshi and Fayyad review the psychological implications of displaced children. Legha and Solages delve into the devastation of the 2010 earthquake in Haiti and the current strategies in developing long-term mental health services. It's hard not to think about health disparities when examining access and quality of psychiatric services. Thus, John-Henderson reviews how our unconscious thoughts and beliefs are important predictors of our behaviors and decisions, which ultimately have an impact on the dynamics of the patient–physician relationship and health-seeking behaviors that may contribute to both adverse and social disparities in health.

Enriching this group of articles includes Song and de Jong's review on the psychological implications of child soldiers in particular. Malhotra and Padhy then provide an overview of the basic challenges in providing child and adolescent psychiatric services in low-resource countries in general. And Srabstein carefully examines the global implications of bullying and other forms of maltreatment. This article highlights the impact of migration and the lack of psychiatric resources.

To round out the series, Latif, Yeatermeyer, Horne, and Beriwal provide a glimpse into the aftermath of nuclear disasters and the impact of such disasters on children and families. Finally, Cullins and Mian focus their article on how culture impacts every level of care—from early identification to prevention and intervention. Cullins and Mian go on to suggest ways to utilize cultural awareness as a strength and treatment innovation.

The field of study of global mental health is quite vast. Thus, unfortunately, space precludes some subject areas from being included in this collection. We hope that this issue on global mental health lays the groundwork for future issues devoted to this important topic. With that said, we are deeply grateful to the contributors to this issue and their commitment, diligence, and expertise. The work that has been done is fascinating, and we are truly inspired and eager to see what more will come. Thank you to all the authors for your extraordinary work. And, thank you to our phenomenal publisher, Elsevier, and the consulting editor, Harsh K. Trivedi, MD.

Paramjit T. Joshi, MD
111 Michigan Avenue NW
Floor 2.5 West–Suite 700
Washington, DC 20010, USA

Lisa M. Cullins, MD
111 Michigan Avenue
Washington, DC 20010, USA

E-mail addresses:
pjoshi@childrensnational.org (P.T. Joshi)
LCullins@childrensnational.org (L.M. Cullins)

Partnering for the World's Children

Why Collaborations Are Important

Paramjit T. Joshi, MD[a,*], Bennett L. Leventhal, MD[b], Joaquin Fuentes, MD[c]

KEYWORDS

• Children • Mental health • Global • Psychiatric disorders • Collaboration

KEY POINTS

- Most psychiatric disorders have their onset in childhood and adolescence when prevention and early intervention can prevent a lifetime of suffering, disability and stigma.
- We share in a global responsibility to transcend cultural and political boundaries to identify childhood-onset psychiatric illness as an international public health crisis.
- The often intertwined contributions of psychosocial, economic, political, cultural, religious, and community variables have an enormous psychological impact on the lives of children and both their physical and mental health.
- Today's problems of poverty and violence will never subside unless we invest in the physical, mental, and emotional development of the next generations.
- We are now in the unique position of having potentially increased the scientific knowledge through research to start addressing these issues in a comprehensive way.
- We must be able to collaborate with colleagues across the world to pursue common goals.

Conflicts: None (P.T. Joshi); Research Funds: Roche, NIH (NIH grant #: 1R01ES021462-01 [PI: Young-Shin Kim, MD, PhD]); Consultant: Janssen (B.L. Leventhal); Research Support: Eli Lilly and Co., Janssen, Shire, Roche, Public Agencies (Spain); Consultant: Eli Lilly and Co., Janssen, Shire, Public Agencies (Spain); Speakers Bureau: Eli Lilly and Co., Shire, Medice; In-Kind Services: Eli Lilly and Co., Janssen, Shire (J. Fuentes Biggi).

[a] Department of Psychiatry & Behavioral Sciences, Children's National Medical Center, George Washington University School of Medicine, 111 Michigan Avenue Northwest, Floor 2.5 West, Suite 700, Washington, DC 20010, USA; [b] Child & Adolescent Psychiatry, Department of Psychiatry, Langley Porter Psychiatric Institute, University of California San Francisco, Box 0984-CAS, Room LP-152, 401 Parnassus Avenue, San Francisco, CA 94143-0984, USA; [c] Child & Adolescent Psychiatry, Policlínica Gipuzkoa, Paseo de Miramón 174, Donostia-San Sebastián 20014, Spain

* Corresponding author.

E-mail address: pjoshi@childrensnational.org

Child Adolesc Psychiatric Clin N Am 24 (2015) 659–677

http://dx.doi.org/10.1016/j.chc.2015.06.001 **childpsych.theclinics.com**

1056-4993/15/$ – see front matter

INTRODUCTION

Today's world finds few places in which children can live in peace, free from violence, deprivation, strife, and hardship; a sad reality. These youth, children, and adolescents of the world, are our future and yet we are permitting them to be exposed and vulnerable to the worst perils of our times.[1] Each and every day millions of children globally are deprived of their right to live in safety, with adequate food, water, shelter, education, and health care, as well as the chance to be reared in caring and loving families with supportive community environments. Daily, children in every corner of the world face the possibility of being kidnapped, killed, orphaned, abandoned, neglected, and/or abused. The reasons are manifold: political, environmental, economic, psychosocial, physical, and even medical or psychiatric illness in their caregivers. And, because of the impoverishment of many families, as well as the disruption of traditional family structures, an increasing number of children have to fend for themselves on the streets. Although the reasons are well known or even understood, there is still no organized move to end this tragedy for our children. The most recent World Health Organization (WHO) Atlas report suggests that the number of children and adolescents facing significant adversity is growing at an alarming rate, and that increasing numbers of children are at risk of deprivation, damaged health, developmental disruption, and premature death.[2] With such a severe, chronic problem, the question becomes: Who will stand up for the world's children?"

BACKGROUND

Mental health is but one part of a child's overall health, development, and ability to learn. The developing brain is a fragile part of each child's body that depends on physical and emotional sustenance from caregivers and the environment. According to the National Institute of Mental Health (NIMH), in the United States, at any point in time, 1 in 5 children has a diagnosable mental disorder and 1 in 10 suffers from a psychiatric illness that is severe enough to impair how they function at home, school and/or in the community.[3,4] The vast majority of psychiatric illnesses appear in childhood and adolescence (50% by age 14 years and 75% by age 24), but the average lag time between the onset of symptoms and the initiation of treatment is 8 to 10 years, even though it has been demonstrated that early diagnosis and intervention for these disorders will impact their prevalence and course, as well as the level of impairment in adult life.[3,4] If children are not screened and treated, these childhood-onset psychiatric disorders persist and contribute to a cycle of school failure, poor employment opportunities, poverty, and suffering that will then affect their descendants.

Children and youth with untreated psychiatric illness have more difficulties in school, more involvement with the criminal justice system, and fewer stable and long-term placements in the child welfare system than do their peers. Although psychiatric disorders impact children from all types of families and at all economic levels, there are certain conditions that can increase the needs for mental health services. Many of the world's children are subject to the most significant of these conditions: living in poverty, witnessing violence, or having a parent who suffers from depression. There are well-researched associations between socioeconomic status and indices of both physical and mental health.[5,6] We need to seize all opportunities to improve health care for millions of children around the world, and we must be able to collaborate, remain organized, and share common goals, so we can speak with one voice on the world stage.

Often, because of the trauma and turmoil in their lives, children and youth in the child welfare and juvenile justice systems have a higher prevalence of psychiatric disorder than do children in the general population. Being a victim of abuse and neglect, being removed from one's family, or living in multiple foster homes can each separately lead to mental health problems; when experienced together, these circumstances multiply the risk for developmental disruption and psychiatric illness. In the United States, considered by most to be a "first world" country, 50% of children in the child welfare system have mental health problems and, in the juvenile justice system, 67% of youth have a diagnosable psychiatric disorder.[7,8]

In the decade to come, we will experience continued population growth worldwide (although at a slower rate compared with the recent past) and with this will come an increasing global need for mental health care for our children and their families. Health care is changing worldwide and we need to ask difficult though important questions of ourselves so that we are better prepared for the future as child and adolescent psychiatrists: What will the delivery of mental health services look like in the near future? Will the treatments be evidence-based? How much will services cost and will our patients be able to afford them? Will our patients get better and how will these outcomes be measured? As child and adolescent psychiatrists, we are uniquely qualified to integrate knowledge about human behavior and development from biological, psychological, familial, social, and cultural perspectives with scientific, humanistic, and collaborative approaches to the diagnosis, treatment, and promotion of mental health in children and adolescents. But, what will be the unique role of child and adolescent psychiatry in the new health care systems?

The Rights of Children

The WHO Mental Health Action Plan 2013–2020 establishes human rights as one of the basic cross-cutting principles for their approved mental health comprehensive plan.[9] It is now well-established that children have rights that entitle them to family-based care, protection, and a fair chance in life. Each child must be loved, protected, and respected[10]; and every child must have the opportunity for an education and access to comprehensive medical care, including psychiatric and psychological services.

SUMMARY OF THE UNITED NATIONS CONVENTION ON THE RIGHTS OF THE CHILD

In 1989, governments worldwide promised all children the same rights by adopting the United Nations (UN) Convention on the Rights of the Child, also known as the CRC or UNCRC.[11] The Convention was intended to change the way children are viewed and treated. It is the most complete statement of children's rights in history. The Convention describes not only rights but also what a child needs to survive, grow, and live up to their potential. These rights and needs apply equally to every child, no matter who they are or where they live. All UN member states, except the United Sates, have ratified the CRC. The UNCRC is charged with ensuring that the Convention is properly observed by the countries that have signed it. The Convention has 54 articles in total. Articles 43 to 54 speak to how adults and governments must work together to ensure that all children's rights are being honored. The following is the list of the Articles that pertain to children[11]:

Article 1
  Definition of the child
  Everyone younger than 18 has all the rights in the Convention.

Article 2
  Without discrimination

The Convention applies to all children, whatever their ethnicity, gender, religion, abilities, whatever they think or say, and no matter what type of family they come from.

Article 3

Best interests of the child

The best interests of the child must be a top priority in all actions concerning children.

Article 4

Protection of rights

Governments must do all they can to fulfill the rights of every child.

Article 5

Parental guidance

Governments must respect the rights and responsibilities of parents to guide and advise their children so that, as they grow, they learn to apply their rights properly.

Article 6

Survival and development

Every child has the right to life. Governments must do all they can to ensure that children survive and grow up healthy.

Article 7

Registration, name, nationality, care

All children have the right to a legally registered name and nationality, as well as the right to know and, as far as possible, to be cared for by their parents.

Article 8

Preservation of identity

Governments must respect and protect a child's identity and prevent the child's name, nationality, or family relationships from being changed unlawfully. If a child has been illegally denied part of his or her identity, governments must act quickly to protect and assist the child to reestablish his or her identity.

Article 9

Separation from parents

Children must not be separated from their parents unless it is in the best interests of the child (for example, in cases of abuse or neglect). A child must be given the chance to express his or her views when decisions about parental responsibilities are being made. Every child has the right to stay in contact with both parents, unless this might harm the child.

Article 10

Family reunification

Governments must respond quickly and sympathetically if a child or the child's parents apply to live together in the same country. If a child's parents live apart in different countries, the child has the right to visit both of them.

Article 11

Kidnapping and trafficking

Governments must take steps to prevent children being taken out of their own country illegally or being prevented from returning.

Article 12

Respect for the views of the child

All children have the right to say what they think in all matters affecting them, and to have their views taken seriously.

Article 13

Freedom of expression

Every child must be free to say what he or she thinks and to seek and receive information of any kind as long as it is within the law.

Article 14

Freedom of thought, belief, and religion

All children have the right to think and believe what they want and also to practice their religion, as long as they are not stopping other people from enjoying their rights. Governments must respect the rights of parents to give their children guidance about this right.

Article 15

Freedom of association

Every child has the right to meet with other children and young people and to join groups and organizations, as long as this does not stop other people from enjoying their rights.

Article 16

Right to privacy

Every child has the right to privacy. The law should protect the child's private, family, and home life.

Article 17

Access to information from mass media

Every child has the right to reliable information from the mass media. Television, radio, newspapers, and other media should provide information that children can understand. Governments must help protect children from materials that could harm them.

Article 18

Parental responsibilities; state assistance

Both parents share responsibility for bringing up their child and should always consider what is best for the child. Governments must help parents by providing services to support them, especially if the child's parents work.

Article 19

Protection from all forms of violence

Governments must do all they can to ensure that children are protected from all forms of violence, abuse, neglect, and mistreatment by their parents or anyone else who looks after them.

Article 20

Children deprived of a family

If a child cannot be looked after by his or her family, governments must make sure that the child is looked after properly by people who respect the child's religion, culture, and language.

Article 21

Adoption

If a child is adopted, the first concern must be what is best for the child. The same protection and standards should apply whether the child is adopted in the country in which the child was born or in another country.

Article 22

Refugee children

If a child is a refugee or seeking refuge, governments must ensure that he or she has the same rights as any other child. Governments must help in trying to reunite child refugees with their parents. When this is not possible, the child should be given protection.

Article 23

Children with disabilities

A child with a disability has the right to live a full and decent life in conditions that promote dignity, independence, and an active role in the community. Governments must do all they can to provide free care and assistance to children with disabilities.

Article 24

Health and health services

Every child has the right to the best possible health. Governments must provide good-quality health care, clean water, nutritious food, and a clean environment so that children can stay healthy. Richer countries must help poorer countries achieve this.

Article 25

Review of treatment in care

If a child has been placed away from home (in care, hospital, or custody, for example), he or she has the right to a regular check of his or her treatment and conditions of care.

Article 26

Social security

Governments must provide extra money for the children of families in need.

Article 27

Adequate standard of living

Every child has the right to a standard of living that is good enough to meet his or her physical, social, and mental needs. Governments must help families that cannot afford to provide this.

Article 28

Right to education

Every child has the right to an education. Primary education must be free. Secondary education must be available to every child. Discipline in schools must respect children's human dignity. Wealthy countries must help poorer countries achieve this.

Article 29

Goals of education

Education must develop every child's personality, talents, and abilities to the full. It must encourage children's respect for human rights, as well as respect for their parents, their own and other cultures, and the environment.

Article 30

Children of minorities

Every child has the right to learn and use the language, customs, and religion of his or her family, whether or not these are shared by most of the people in the country in which the child lives.

Article 31

Leisure, play, and culture

Every child has the right to relax, play, and join in a wide range of cultural and artistic activities.

Article 32

Child labor

Governments must protect children from work that is dangerous or might harm their health or education.

Article 33

Drug abuse

Governments must protect children from the use of illegal drugs.

Article 34

Sexual exploitation

Governments must protect children from sexual abuse and exploitation.

Article 35

Abduction

Governments must ensure that children are not abducted or sold.

Article 36

Other forms of exploitation

Governments must protect children from all other forms of exploitation that might harm them.

Article 37

Detention

No child shall be tortured or suffer other cruel treatment or punishment. A child shall only ever be arrested or put in prison as a last resort and for the shortest possible time. Children must not be put in a prison with adults and they must be able to keep in contact with their family.

Article 38

War and armed conflicts: see "Optional protocols"

Governments must do everything they can to protect and care for children affected by war. Governments must not allow children younger than 15 to take part in war or join the armed forces.

Article 39
Rehabilitation of child victims
Children neglected, abused, exploited, or tortured or who are victims of war must receive special help to help them recover their health, dignity, and self-respect.

Article 40
Juvenile justice
A child accused or guilty of breaking the law must be treated with dignity and respect. Children have the right to help from a lawyer and a fair trial that takes account of their age or situation. The child's privacy must be respected at all times.

Article 41
Respect for better national standards
If the laws of a particular country protect children better than the articles of the Convention, then those laws must stay.

Article 42
Knowledge of rights
Governments must make the Convention known to children and adults.

OPTIONAL ADDITIONS

In 2000, the UN General Assembly adopted 2 optional additions to strengthen the Convention. One required governments to increase the minimum age for recruitment into the armed forces from 15 years and to ensure that members of their armed forces younger than 18 did not take part in armed conflict. The other provides detailed requirements for governments to end the sexual exploitation and abuse of children. It also protects children from being sold for nonsexual purposes, such as other forms of forced labor, illegal adoption, and organ donation.

There even needs to be a bill of rights for children that speaks to the challenges facing our youth and their parents and caregivers. And, although each of these declarations seems self-evident, despite the guarantees of so many countries, the rights of children are routinely ignored or flagrantly violated. All children are vulnerable, but it is those with disabilities and, especially, the high-prevalence, high-impact disabilities associated with psychiatric illness that are at the greatest risk.

A CALL TO ACTION

The stakes are high. Although many challenges face our developing youth, psychiatric disorders represent perhaps the most common, high-impact, chronic problem for which there are the most limited resources. One in 5 children either currently or perhaps as many as 50% will have a disorder at some point during their lifetime, many of which will be seriously debilitating.[3,4] The seriousness of this situation is amplified because fewer than 20% of those affected will receive appropriate treatment, and virtually all of those who receive care will be in the highly developed nations. This means that it is more likely than not that children in the developing world will receive no care at all, and the consequences are severe.

- More youth and young adults continue to die from suicide than from all natural causes combined. It is argued whether suicide is the second or third most common cause of death. For example, according to WHO, suicide is the second leading cause of death among those 15 to 29 years old, and 75% of global suicides occur in low-income and middle-income countries.[12] This is a specious argument. We know suicide is much more common that all other medical illnesses and is only possibly exceeded by accidents and homicide. Ninety percent of those who die by suicide have a psychiatric disorder that was diagnosed before death. And, despite recent advances in treatment, we have not yet been able to make much progress in reducing the rates of youth suicide, except in countries that have strong laws restricting access to guns, like Australia, which must also be noted to have a strong multifaceted approach to youth suicide.[13]
  - Approximately 50% of students younger than 14 with a psychiatric illness will drop out of school, with members of racial and ethnic minority groups dropping out at higher rates, as do those from low-income families, from single-parent households, and from families in which one or both parents also did not complete high school.[4] This all suggests that powerful psychosocial factors interact with the presence of illness to place youth at risk.
  - Seventy percent of youth in juvenile justice systems have at least one psychiatric diagnosis.
  - The longer patients with mental illness stay ill, the more expensive it is to manage (this loss includes cost of care and lack of productivity in work/society).

Timely access, standards of care, and perceptions about mental illness remain challenges. An 8-year to 10-year delay between the onset of symptoms and intervention is simply unacceptable: imagine the international outrage if this were the case for cancer. Time and resources invested in the child's care, both early in life and early in the course of illness, will have a significant impact on their future health, quality of life, and cost of care. Thus, we must prioritize timely, early, multidisciplinary assessments for children. This sort of collaboration and attention to details and evidence-based care will create a brighter future for our patients and their families.

In recent times, there have been very visible tragedies involving our youth. All-too-frequent examples include shootings in the United States, the kidnapping of girls in Nigeria, and selling of children for labor or sex trafficking in Southeast Asia, to mention a few of the many. These have included all manner of violence and privation, and, after each of these, it has been suggested that long-standing mental health problems either contributed to or will be the consequences of these awful events. After each of these events, there is a momentary resolve by leaders and citizens to bring the issues of the rights of children and their mental health back to the national and international stage; yet, with the 24-hour news cycle, these stories quickly disappear from the prominent media outlets, and little has been done systemically. The underlying problems are not addressed, and children remain at risk and in jeopardy. These stories that produce media frenzies are but the tip of the iceberg, as millions of youth around the world struggle with psychiatric illnesses with no hope of help. How many will have their educational, social, and vocational development disrupted or, worse, commit suicide because they did not get needed services? Indeed, why in the twenty-first century are we even asking this question?

Children's mental health has been identified for too long as one of the most underserved areas in all of medicine. It is a discipline that is understaffed, underfunded, poorly reimbursed, and poorly understood from a research perspective. The vast majority of the mental health professionals are in developed countries, such as the United States. Even in the United States, uneven distribution and lack of access means that only 25% of children in need receive services and, even then, the delays are inordinate and the services often inadequate. Children throughout the world are even worse off. There are countries like India with less than a dozen trained child and adolescent psychiatrists, and some countries have none at all. WHO reports that the number of general psychiatrists, not child psychiatrists, is 30 per 100,000 in Switzerland, 1 per 100,000 in Turkey, and in Liberia the figure is 0.06 mental health professionals per 100,000. Equally shocking is that many countries do not even have public policy related to children's mental health.[2]

It is often said that one of the reasons for the lack of appropriate children's mental health care is the absence of science about the causes and treatments of childhood-onset psychiatric disorders, but the data are to the contrary. Although blood tests are not yet available, the neurobiology and genetics of childhood-onset disorders are becoming increasingly clear. As with other areas of medicine, despite the lack of specific etiologies for clinical syndromes, there are evidence-based, safe, and effective pharmacologic and psychosocial/environmental interventions for the most prevalent of disorders. Because psychiatric illness is very much a "childhood" issue that greatly affects a child's overall health, development, learning abilities, and future competitiveness in society, it is time for these advances to be applied to children throughout the world.

More recently, with mounting evidence from studies such as the Milliman report on adults with mental health disorders, integrating general medical and psychiatric care (integrated care) is essential, as it results not only in improved outcome but also measurable financial savings.[5] On a purely economic basis, early identification and effective treatment of childhood-onset psychiatric disorders is cost-effective and results in decreased lifetime care costs, as well as increased earning potential for the individual. In other pediatric chronic conditions, such as obesity, asthma, and diabetes, early detection and intervention have produced a positive effect on patients' health as they enter adulthood and have led to improved lifetime outcomes. For psychiatric illnesses, the data are very similar: early recognition and timely intervention can delay or prevent the onset of psychopathology and result in faster, more complete recovery. It also can decrease the frequency and severity of relapses. A 33-year follow-up study of children with attention-deficit/hyperactivity disorder (ADHD) demonstrated the value of early treatment. Children who did not receive intervention experienced an increased likelihood of incarceration and early death in adulthood compared with matched controls.[14] These and other findings highlight the importance of extended monitoring and treatment of children with ADHD.[14] In another study, children at high risk for psychosis who received early identification and treatment did not develop a psychotic disorder, demonstrating that the course of psychosis is not fixed, as was previously believed.[15]

In June 2014, President Obama held a White House Summit on Mental Health, the first in 15 years, focusing on pediatric psychiatric disorders. In a subsequent national meeting of government policy makers, NIMH leaders, and leaders of child and adolescent psychiatry and pediatrics, there was an attempt to find solutions for how best to address the pressing needs of individuals experiencing a psychiatric illness in the United States. This was prompted by a public outcry in light of a spate of horrific public massacres. And, once again, with the decline in media attention, came a decline in this effort, as well. How can this happen when so many recognized that the time for leadership is now and that there must be a change in the conversation about mental health? The discussions have ended once again. This means that we are failing both the children who perish in such tragedies and those who we are fortunate enough to still have in our care. There is a social and moral imperative to support the 1 in 5 children who need care now. Physically and mentally healthy children are more likely to become physically and mentally healthy adults. These children will grow up and enter our armed forces, our intelligence communities, our workforces, and our governments.[16] This demand is not just in North America, but for children on each and every continent.

CHALLENGES AND OPPORTUNITIES

President Obama's New Freedom Commission on Mental Health concluded that "no other illness has damaged so many children so seriously." This is true for the United States and around the world. Given these challenges and opportunities, the following initiatives are critically required.

Providing Timely Access to Care

Children are rapidly developing, so that even a modest developmental disruption can have wide-ranging impacts on later life. A missed few weeks of school due to depression, anxiety, or inattention can mean a lifetime of trouble with reading, writing, or mathematics. Time and resources invested in a child's care at or before the onset of symptoms will result in a quantifiable improvement in future health, quality of life, and cost of care. To meet this challenge, primary care providers must have better training for screening and initiating care. The primary care providers also need back-up from many more child and adolescent psychiatrists, psychologists, social workers, nurse practitioners, and others who must be trained and available to devote the necessary time and attention to the care of children.

Developing Standards of Care

"Mental health" is a term that is far too vague, and has been allowed to be too broadly defined. It is time to think about "psychiatric illnesses," which, like other medical disorders, involve an organ system that interacts with the environment in health and disease. Psychiatric illnesses are disorders of brain function that interfere with cognition (including memory and learning), emotion, and behavior. In child and adolescent psychiatry, these symptoms must be examined in a developmental context. As with developmental medical disorders, it takes a multidisciplinary team working closely together to provide adequate evaluations. There is an ample evidence base to set universal standards for these assessments and treatments, as well as the standards for training to participate in the care of children with psychiatric disorders. Establishing these universal standards for care and training will go a long way in leveling the playing field when it comes to the evidence-based treatments.

Stop the Stigma and Discrimination

Stigma and bias are powerful forces that not only lead to the abuse of individuals with psychiatric disorders, but it is even more ominous how they shape national and international policies on availability and accessibility to services. Barriers based on bias and stigma must be removed, and psychiatric illnesses must be placed on equal footing with all other medical conditions that deserve the attention of health and public health systems. For the many conditions that require acute care, patients and families should be offered not only access, but also encouragement and support for care. For many with chronic psychiatric illness, they should receive services for their chronic psychiatric condition in the same manner and integrated with the care received by others with similar chronic disorders. Stigma not only leads to abuse of patients with psychiatric disorders but makes them feel bad about themselves, a reflection of poor societal practices and governmental policies that foster fear, contempt, and hatred for children and families faced with the challenges of psychiatric illnesses. Psychiatric illness is the leprosy of the modern era. This bias is a global problem, with cultural, political, and geographic ramifications that must be addressed openly and clearly at the highest levels.

Performing Clinical and Translational Research

Rapid advances in neuroscience and genetics open great clinical and translational research opportunities, including the possibility of identifying molecular targets and pathways for innovative pharmacotherapeutics, as well as the use of biomarkers that allow for earlier detection and provide endpoints for intervention trials. Technological breakthroughs during the past few years have helped us to understand, identify, and intervene in many medical issues before they manifest symptoms. Therefore, any discussion of the biological basis of psychiatric disorders must include genetics and behavioral neuroscience. Indeed, we are beginning to fit new pieces into the puzzle of how genetic mutations influence brain development. In 2009, NIMH launched the Research Domain Criteria (RDoC) project, which is developing a mental disorders classification system for research, based more on underlying causes than on symptoms. It is hoped that the RDoC project will go beyond our current disorder classification system to look at the behavior systems and fundamental brain circuits that cut across many disorders.[17]

Fostering Models of Cross-Disciplinary Integration

The first principle stated by the WHO Mental Health Action Plan (2013–2020) is "equity." Equity speaks to the critical need for universal health coverage.[2] The time has come to ensure a cross-disciplinary mental health assessment for children, spanning pediatrics, psychology/psychiatry, social work, physical medicine and rehabilitation, neuropsychology, and neurology. We must foster collaborations among specialists from neurology, psychiatry, genetics, and behavioral disciplines, with seamless integration between clinical and academic spheres. In addition, partnerships with nonmedical specialties and stakeholders are crucial, as well as clearly defined roles for such entities as the offices of education, employment, judiciary, housing, social, and other relevant public and private sectors. Further, the payment system needs to support such a collaborative approach to care.

Increasing Funding for Research on Psychiatric Disorders

Enhanced funding for research is needed, and we need to advocate for and invest in our future research efforts. We need to take advantage of breakthroughs in genetics, the launch of the Brain Research through Advancing Innovative Neurotechnologies (BRAIN) initiative supported by President Obama, and the progress with the Human Connectome Program under way at NIMH.[18,19] It is necessary to foster public/private partnerships in securing much needed funding that is both sustained and sustainable to advance the field.

Funding and Enforcement of Mental Health Parity with Other Medical Illnesses Is Essential

There must be the clear expectation that mental health services are an integral part of the care system for children and adolescents. They not only must be created with the same vigor and quality as other health care but also be given similar resources to provide this essential element of health care for children and adolescents.

The Child and Adolescent Mental Health Atlas highlights the gaps in mental health care for children around the world and proposes steps for how to bridge these gaps.[2] The WHO, Department of Mental Health and Substance Abuse, supported the development of the Atlas project. The project provides systematic information on country resources for mental health program development, including policy availability, professional resources, and mechanisms for financing services. The Child and Adolescent Mental Health Atlas is a part of this series of publications.[2] The work on the Child and Adolescent Mental Health Atlas was carried out by WHO, in close collaboration with the World Psychiatric Association (WPA) Presidential Global Program on Child Mental Health and in collaboration with the International Association for Child and Adolescent Psychiatry and Allied Professions (IACAPAP). The WPA has a history of long-standing and fruitful collaboration with WHO in the area of mental health.

The Atlas proposes the following urgent needs.

Enhanced Information

There is a need for enhanced information on child and adolescent mental health disorders and the resources available to provide care. The Atlas recommends the implementation of WHO's Assessment Instrument for Mental Health Systems (WHO-AIMS) that can assist in this process.[20]

Policy

The Atlas urges ministers of health and other interested parties in all countries to help bridge the gaps in policies around children's mental health issues with the new *WHO Child and Adolescent Mental Health Policies and Plans Manual*, which is a great resource providing a guidance in developing policy and establishing appropriate governance.

Training

Atlas has shown that there are gaps in mental health training among primary care providers, educators, and others. Training for these professionals would certainly enhance access and resources and allow for early identification and intervention, which is a very much desired goal.

Financing

The need for sustained and sustainable financing of services is crucial. Such services cannot be sustained indefinitely on funding and/or grants from nongovernmental organizations and the like. If governments around the world are serious about providing mental health services to their children, they have a moral obligation to step forward and provide the funding for sustained and quality services and provide parity between adult and child services.

WITH WHOM DO WE PARTNER AND WHY IS PARTNERING IMPORTANT?

International Organizations

It is vitally important that all child and adolescent psychiatric organizations around the world come together and form strong collaborations around common themes. Although each organization has its own resources, meetings, policy statements, and advocacy efforts to strengthen the common purpose, it will be advantageous for each to support the other and, when possible, share resources and globally promote identical policies for children's mental health. In the end, there really is power in numbers. If organizations such as the American Academy of Child and Adolescent

Psychiatry, IACAPAP, WPA, Economic and Social Commission for Asia and the Pacific, and Asian Society for Child and Adolescent Psychiatry and Allied Professions, to name a few, will partner on behalf of our children, we will improve children's rights, as well as make strides in early identification and intervention for psychiatric illnesses that affect children. Together, we can more effectively advocate for the proper and fair allocation of resources, promote evidence-based treatments, and support investment in research efforts to uncover the etiologic substrates of disorders, along with better and more effective treatments.

Each of the individual organizations and professional societies has good ideas. Each has been creative in their own way. By sharing this creativity and strategies that have proven successful, we each do not have to start over. No one organization can or should try to do it all or all by themselves. As an example, it will be in everyone's best interest to list the rich and extraordinary resources available on our Web sites and provide links in one place that connects all of the other resources available from other child and adolescent psychiatry organizations, so that these can be readily accessed by anyone across the globe.

It is our responsibility to be able to provide for our children in a holistic manner and provide a safe living environment that encompasses a multifocal approach so that children can reach their potential and have a real opportunity to grow and develop socially, emotionally, and physically so that they can become independent and productive members of society and be able to contribute to life in a meaningful manner. A special liaison also must be established with international agencies responding to humanitarian emergencies (including isolated, repeated, or continuing conflict, violence, or disasters).

Pediatricians and primary care physicians have an important role to play in identifying and initiating treatment of mental health disorders, especially given the documented shortage of child and adolescent psychiatrists.[21–23] Yet, many challenges remain to ensure that pediatricians and primary care physicians have the skills, knowledge and time to properly identify and treat mental health concerns and to make appropriate referrals.[24,25] A collaborative "medical home" model is needed to address access to mental health care. Moreover, a fundamental change in our approach to the diagnosis and treatment of childhood psychiatric illness is needed. Psychiatric illness does not generally arise solely from family stresses or environmental influences. There is evidence that discernible molecular aberrations in genetics, brain structure, function, and cellular signaling and connectivity can place individuals at increased risk for mental illness from early childhood.[26] Only after these endogenous alterations are identified, through further research studies, can mental conditions be assessed and treated as medical conditions. They then can be approached and "cured" by personalized, precise treatments, rather than lumped into misleading categories, resulting in nonspecific, often ineffective treatments.

It is a major challenge to integrate basic mental health care into primary care; however, this will be a core element of getting mental health parity right. It can be done well, improving health and reducing costs, but barriers must be addressed. We know that most children are treated by their pediatricians or other primary care practitioners rather than by child and adolescent psychiatrists. Improving basic mental health care in the primary care setting is a great need, opportunity, and sensible goal. We have the responsibility to embrace and take the lead in moving this forward. At the same time, we must also ensure cross-disciplinary assessment for children. Furthermore, standardization and integration of mental health care, such as electronic medical records and integrated databases, will be important.

Currently, we are taking care of organ systems instead of the total patient. The future lies in transforming the understanding and treatment of mental illnesses through basic and clinical research; paving the way for prevention, recovery, and cure by looking at the pathophysiology, predictive biomarkers, and preemptive interventions; and viewing mental illnesses as developmental disorders.[27]

The time has come to shift the dialogue about children's mental health. The different strategies that we have been using have not worked. In medical school, we were taught to think backwards: to diagnose things after they occur, to cure things after they happen. But what if we flip this model by looking forward, anticipating, and intervening before the symptoms appear? Ultimately, it is not just about keeping our children healthy, but also about creating a society of healthy adults. As pediatricians and child and adolescent psychiatrists, we are already trained to think forward. We think developmentally by asking, for example, What do we expect at 2 months, 4 months, 8 months, and 2 years? This is the approach needed to ensure that we are capturing the mental health needs of our children.[27]

Pediatricians have a critical role in the identification children at risk, including the roles of parents and caregivers in this process. Not only must the child be assessed, but also the family and other elements in the environment. For example, we know that women frequently experience postpartum depression, as well as depression in general. Because maternal depression can have severe adverse impacts on the developing child, appropriate care of the children includes screening mothers who may suffer from depression or other mental health problems. Children whose mothers are depressed have a higher prevalence of mental health problems.[28] Low-income mothers with young children have shown rates of depression ranging as high as 40% to 60%, and a large percentage of these mothers have never spoken to any medical professional about their depressive symptoms.[28] Maternal depression threatens attachment and bonding, which are psychological processes critical to an infant's development. Living with a mother suffering from depression also can have negative effects on a child's cognitive and social-emotional development, behavior, and language acquisition. These problems do not just impact infants, but also can impact older children: behavior disorders, attachments disorders, depression, and other mood disorders in childhood and adolescence can occur more often in children of mothers with major depression.[29,30] The importance of maternal health to a child's development, has led the American Academy of Pediatrics (AAP) to expect pediatricians to routinely screen mothers for depression during prenatal and postpartum visits to heath care providers. As the AAP notes, treating a child includes optimizing that child's healthy development and healthy family functioning.

Role of the Medical Home

The rapid expansion of the medical home model is changing the face of medical care for children. The basic notion is that all medically relevant care is provided in a single setting. Pediatricians and/or other primary care providers will not only be adjacent to but, rather, integrated with the rest of the health care providers, ranging from dentists to nutritionists and mental health professionals. The medical home provides excellent care that is accessible, family-centered, comprehensive, continuous, coordinated, compassionate, and culturally competent while including concerted outreach to families, with an emphasis on the cultural context, and integration with schools and recreational, vocational, and other community services.

Schools

In almost every country, schools (partnering with health and mental health organizations) are being seriously considered to be the largest provider of mental health services to children, among children who receive mental health services. Because the overwhelming majority of children attend school, schools are an ideal location to identify children with mental health needs and provide them with appropriate services. Students and parents also are familiar with school facilities and staff, which helps lessen the stigma of seeking help for mental health issues. These children also are more likely to drop out or fail out of school: up to 14% of students with mental health problems receive mostly poor or failing grades and up to 44% drop out of high school. In the course of a school year, children with mental health problems may miss as many as 18 to 22 days of school, so if the mental health services are provided at school this can be reduced. School-based mental health programs should be expanded to reach all students in every country across the globe.[31]

Communities

Early intervention is another critical concept and includes both community-based services and transition services. Children live, play, and go to school in a community, so another important approach is to think about how to enrich the community to serve the children. Families and communities are becoming increasingly sophisticated in understanding health. Many health and health-related services are now routinely delivered in the community. Family and children must be the focus, and family support is critical. The community-based team can include family counseling, social services, sibling projects, primary care and other medical providers, the school, and religious and spiritual supports. Other facets of family support are respite services, educational workshops, group sessions, parent-to-parent outreach, and a parent library of resources. Prevention efforts and solid support are most effective when they involve stakeholders and local community partners. This community approach must consider empowering children, adolescents, and families with mental disorders and psychosocial disabilities.

SUMMARY

There are few human tragedies that stir sympathy and concern more deeply than seeing children suffer for any reason. However, the often-intertwined contributions of psychosocial, economic, political, cultural, religious, and community variables have come to be appreciated as confounding factors having an enormous psychological impact on the lives of children and both their physical and mental health. Children are not born to hate, hurt others, or take revenge. What happens, then, in places like the Congo where boys are recruited to become soldiers? How do stone-throwing youngsters become suicide bombers? How do youngsters here at home in the United States take a gun to school and indiscriminately shoot at their classmates and teachers? Why do children younger and younger with every passing generation want to die by suicide? These are but a few of the vexing questions that beg answers arising when analyzing the effects of unmet mental health needs.

Today's problems of poverty and violence will never subside unless we invest in the physical, mental, and emotional development of the next generations. All of us continue to struggle to make sense of what happened on September 11th, and what continues to happen in places like the Middle East, Afghanistan, Tibet, Central Africa, and other parts of the world. It is hoped that our experience of shared vulnerability and common purpose can be productively incorporated into the work we do with children and families all over the world. We are now in the unique position of having potentially increased the scientific knowledge through research to start addressing these issues in a comprehensive way.[32] The work across many disciplines of children's mental health care needs our sincere attention to spur progress on all of the fronts to effectuate the shortcomings in the current approach. Mental health concerns globally are coming out of the shadows at a time of major change in health care, and we need to seize all opportunities to improve health care for millions of children. We need to remain optimistic that together we can all work to advance our field, preserve our identity as child and adolescent psychiatrists, and provide the best care that we can to our patients. To do this, we must be able to collaborate with colleagues across the world, hold hands and pursue common goals and agendas, so we can speak with one voice on behalf of our children.

In the words of the Chilean poet, Gabriela Mistral:

Many things can wait.

The child cannot.

Now is the time

His blood is being formed,

His bones are being made,

His mind is being developed.

To him, we cannot say tomorrow,

His name is today.

REFERENCES

1. Kessler RC, Amminger GP, Aguilar-Gaxiola S, et al. Age of onset of mental disorders: a review of recent literature. Curr Opin Psychiatry 2007;20(4):359–64.
2. WHO: Mental Health Atlas. Geneva, Switzerland: WHO Press; 2011. Available at: www.who.int. Accessed June 02, 2015.
3. National Research Council and Institute of Medicine of the National Academies. Preventing mental, emotional, and behavioral disorders among young people: progress and possibilities. The National Academic Press Consensus Report March 12, 2009.
4. Centers for Disease Control and Prevention. Mental health surveillance among children—United States, 2005–2011. MMWR Surveill Summ 2013;62(Suppl): 1–35. Available at: www.cdc.gov/mmwr/pdf/ss/ss6104.pdf.
5. Economic Impact of Integrated Medical-Behavioral Healthcare. Milliman-Report-Final. Available at: http://us.milliman.com. Accessed August 13, 2013.
6. Foster EM, Connor T. Public cost of better mental health services for children and adolescents. Psychiatr Serv 2005;56:50–5.
7. Costello EJ, Angold A, Burns BJ, et al. The Great Smoky Mountains study of youth. Functional impairment and serious emotional disturbance. Arch Gen Psychiatry 1996;54:1137–43.
8. Merikangas KR, He JP, Burstein M, et al. Lifetime prevalence of mental disorders in U.S. adolescents: results from the National Comorbidity Survey

Replication–Adolescent Supplement (NCS-A). J Am Acad Child Adolesc Psychiatry 2010;49(10):980–9.
9. WHO Mental Health Action Plan 2013-2020 (WHO Press) ISBN: 978 92 4 150602.
10. Carlson M. Child rights and mental health. Child Adolesc Psychiatr Clin N Am 2002;10(4):825–39.
11. UN High Commissioner for Human Rights, 'UN Convention on the Rights of the Child,' UN General Assembly, Geneva. Available at: http://www.unhcr.org. Accessed November 20, 1989.
12. World Health Organization. The global burden of disease—2004 update. Geneva (Switzerland): WHO; 2008. Available at: http://www.who.int/healthinfo/global_burden_disease/2004_report_update/en/.
13. Before it's too late: Report on the inquiry into early intervention programs aimed at reducing youth suicide. Australian Government. 2013. Available at: http://www.health.gov.au/internet/main/publishing.nsf/Content/0B356361B55CEE4ECA257BF0001A8E4D/$File/before.pdf. Accessed February 14, 2015.
14. Klein RG, Mannuzza S, Olazagasti MA, et al. Clinical and functional outcome of childhood ADHD 33 years later. Arch Gen Psychiatry 2012;69(12):1295–303.
15. Agius M, Shah S, Ramkisson R, et al. Three year outcomes of an early intervention for psychosis service as compared with treatment as usual for first psychotic episodes in a standard community mental health team. Preliminary results. Psychiatr Danub 2007;19(1–2):10–9.
16. Joshi PT. Mental health services for children and adolescents: challenges and opportunities [editorial]. JAMA Psychiatry 2014;71(1):17–8.
17. Insel T, Cuthbert B, Garvey M, et al. Research domain criteria (RDoC): toward a new classification framework for research on mental disorders. Am J Psychiatry 2010;167:748–51.
18. The Brain Initiative and Brain Research through advancing innovative neurotechnologies. NIMH.gov. The U.S. Department of Health and Human Services [HHS]. brain@ostp.gov.
19. National Institute of Mental Health Strategic Plan. 2015. Available at: www.nimh.nih.gov. Accessed March 26, 2015.
20. World Health Organization assessment instrument for mental health system (WHO-AIMS) version 2.2. Geneva (Switzerland): World Health Organization; 2005.
21. Thomas CR, Holzer CE. The continuing shortage of child and adolescent psychiatrists. J Am Acad Child Adolesc Psychiatry 2006;45:1023–31.
22. Shatkin JP, Belfer ML. The global absence of child and adolescent mental health policy. Child Adolesc Mental Health 2004;9(3):104–8.
23. The world health report 2001—mental health: new understanding, new hope. Geneva (Switzerland): World Health Organization; 2001.
24. Heneghan A, Garner AS, Storfer-Isser A, et al. Pediatricians' role in providing mental health care for children and adolescents: do pediatricians and child and adolescent psychiatrists agree? J Dev Behav Pediatr 2008;29:262–9.
25. Ross WJ, Chan E, Harris SK, et al. Pediatrician-psychiatrist collaboration to care for children with attention deficit hyperactivity disorder, depression and anxiety. Clin Pediatr 2011;50:37–43.
26. Insel TR. Next generation treatments for mental disorders. Sci Transl Med 2012;4(155):155ps19.
27. Joshi PT. Presidential address: partnering for the world's children. J Am Acad Child Adolesc Psychiatry 2014;53(1):3–8.

28. Lyons-Ruth K, Connell DB, Grunebaum H. Infants at social risk: maternal depression and family support services as mediators of infant development and security of attachment. Child Dev 1990;61:85–98.
29. Lieberman AF, Zeanah CH. Disorders of attachment in infancy. Child Adolesc Psychiatr Clin N Am 1995;4:574–87.
30. NICE Guideline PH40 ("Social & emotional wellbeing: early years"). Available at: https://www.nice.org.uk/guidance/ph40/chapter/appendix-c-the-evidence. Accessed October 24, 2012.
31. Porter GK, Pearson GT, Keenan S, et al. School-based mental health services: a necessity, not a luxury. In: Pumariega AJ, Winters NC, editors. Handbook of community-based systems of care: the new child and adolescent community psychiatry. New York: Jossey-Bass; 2003. p. 250–75.
32. Collins PY, Patel V, Joestl SS, et al. Grand challenges in global mental health. Nature 2011;475:27–30.

Advancing Research to Action in Global Child Mental Health

Anna E. Ordóñez, MD, MAS[a], Pamela Y. Collins, MD, MPH[b,*]

KEYWORDS

• Global mental health research • Research capacity building • Children
• Adolescents • Grand challenges • Child development

KEY POINTS

- Research plays an essential role in global mental health.
- The knowledge and interventions generated by research must be translated to action to achieve public health impact.
- Global research relevant to child and adolescent mental health requires multidisciplinary collaboration and the capacity to conduct research activities that range from basic neuroscience to health policy research.
- Equitable research collaborations can facilitate research capacity building and ensure full participation of high-income country (HIC) and low- and middle-income country (LMIC) researchers to solve problems.

INTRODUCTION

Child and adolescent mental health (CAMH) problems are largely neglected in the wider realm of global public health, and this lack of attention has implications for young people's health, well-being, and longevity. The World Health Organization (WHO) estimates that more than 800,000 people committed suicide in 2012. Suicide is the second leading killer of people aged 15 to 29 years,[1] and in regions of the world where targeted interventions have successfully reduced rates of maternal

The authors have no disclosures.
The viewpoints expressed in this article do not necessarily reflect the views of the National Institute of Mental Health.

[a] Office of Clinical Research, National Institute of Mental Health (NIMH), National Institutes of Health (NIH), Bethesda, Maryland 20892, USA; [b] Office for Research on Disparities and Global Mental Health, National Institute of Mental Health (NIMH), National Institutes of Health (NIH), 6001 Executive Boulevard, Suite 6217, Bethesda, MD 20892, USA
* Corresponding author.
E-mail address: pamela.collins@nih.gov

Child Adolesc Psychiatric Clin N Am 24 (2015) 679–697
http://dx.doi.org/10.1016/j.chc.2015.06.002
1056-4993/15/$ – see front matter Published by Elsevier Inc.
childpsych.theclinics.com

mortality, it is the leading killer of young women aged 15 to 19 years.[2] Within countries, suicide rates differ among subpopulations, and young people in some communities are distinctly vulnerable. A regional analysis of suicide from 1999 to 2009 among Alaska Native and American Indian populations showed particularly high rates among Alaska Native communities and suicide rate among people younger than 44 years was 5 times the suicide rate of White Americans in the United States.[3] In Nunavut, the northernmost territory of Canada, around 65% of suicides among the Inuit population between 1999 and 2014 occurred among people aged 10 to 24 years.[4]

Evidence-based interventions implemented through regional, national, and global suicide prevention plans provide one example of how health systems can use data to generate strategies for control and to stimulate policy responses from decision makers. The WHO's Comprehensive Mental Health Action Plan 2013–2020 sets a global target of 10% reduction in suicides by 2020 across member states and calls for strengthened information systems, evidence, and research on mental health.[5] In the United States, the Prioritized Research Agenda for Suicide Prevention calls for a 20% reduction in suicides over the next 5 years and 40% reduction over the next 10 years.[6] The investigators note, "A research document alone cannot reduce suicide deaths or attempts; rather, its intent is to identify the research needed to guide practice and inform policy decisions across many areas."[6]

These efforts call attention to the role that research can play in supporting and stimulating a public health agenda. Research provides the evidence base for successful interventions, data for monitoring progress, and, over the long run, makes solutions available to complex problems. Globally, research is needed to spur public health action to reduce the mortality and morbidity associated with poor mental health in childhood and adolescence. Children, adolescents, and youth represent more than one-third of the world's population. In 2010, 35.4% of the world's population was aged between 0 and 19 years and 44.3% was aged between 0 and 24 years.[7] In the least developed countries, these populations represent 51.6% and 60.8% of the total population, respectively.

Most mental and substance use disorders begin during childhood and adolescence,[8] with 75% of cases beginning before the age of 25 years in the United States.[9] Developmental disabilities, conduct disorder, attention deficit-hyperactivity disorder, anxiety, and depression confer the greatest burden of disease for children younger than 10 years[10]; these are disabling disorders of youth across continents with vastly different health profiles and remain the leading causes for disability worldwide.[11] At the same time, the periods of infancy, childhood, and adolescence represent opportune times for interventions to reduce risk for mental disorders and enhance social, emotional, and cognitive functioning.[12] Researchers seeking to understand developmental trajectories of brain development and their relationship to mental disorders increasingly view these disorders as neurodevelopmental.[13] Researchers are exploring how changes in neural architecture correspond to developmental stages and respond to contextual and environmental exposures.[12] This work opens the door to better understanding risk and protective factors and to the development of effective multilevel interventions.

Optimizing this research enterprise to ensure global representation has been challenging. The 10/90 research gap, which refers to the inequity in distribution of research investments and activities, highlighted 20 years ago by the Commission on Health Research for Development,[14] is particularly striking in the area of child mental health. Although 90% of the world's children live in developing countries, only 10% of randomized controlled trials testing mental health interventions for children occurred in

LMICs.[15] Even fewer studies address psychosocial and combined interventions for children's mental health problems.[15] Nevertheless, a key function (and challenge) for health systems everywhere is the use of research findings and implementation of research-based interventions for CAMH in routine practice.[16] For these reasons, research is an integral part of the global health system.[17] Developing an agenda and the associated priorities lead this process, followed by financing and resource allocation, research and development, implementation and delivery of services, as well as monitoring and evaluation, while ensuring that means for learning from the knowledge gained are built into the process.[17,18]

In this article, the authors use selected findings from a recent research priority-setting exercise, the Grand Challenges in Global Mental Health, to organize the presentation of priorities for global CAMH research and public health action. The initiative articulates a set of challenges with particular relevance to children and adolescents that, if addressed in a coordinated manner, have the potential to improve outcomes in early child development (ECD) and mental health. For each challenge, the authors describe existing research-informed initiatives with national and global reach that can contribute to solving the challenges, and they also discuss the research capacity building needed to undertake these challenges.

RESEARCH PRIORITY SETTING FOR GLOBAL MENTAL HEALTH

Over the past decade, Grand Challenge initiatives focused on global health priorities have mobilized global cooperation, resource allocation, and research in efforts to solve intractable problems.[19,20] In 2010, the National Institute of Mental Health and partners, including the Global Alliance for Chronic Disease, launched the Grand Challenges in Global Mental Health.[21] The initiative convened more than 400 researchers, clinicians, and advocates from 60 countries to identify priorities for research that, if addressed, could make an impact on the lives of people with mental, neurologic, and substance use disorders worldwide.

Unlike previous priority-setting exercises,[22–24] the initiative identified challenges for HICs and LMICs and focused on mental, neurologic, and substance use disorders. Three rounds of a Delphi procedure, a structured consensus-building process, yielded 40 challenges. The top 25 challenges were categorized across 6 goals that spanned the range of science—from discovery research to policy research.[21] In addition, the following 4 cross-cutting themes emerged from the data:

1. Researchers and decision makers must adopt a life course approach to carry out research and action on these issues.
2. Approaches to mental, neurological, and substance use (MNS) disorders cannot solely be addressed within siloed health care, but must be addressed across the health system and across sectors.
3. Interventions must be evidence based.
4. Context matters—the impact of environmental exposures and experience on risk, resilience, and interventions should be understood.

The authors focus on 5 challenges relevant to CAMH that are associated with Goal B: Advance prevention and implementation of early interventions (**Box 1**).

Challenge 1: Support Community Environments that Promote Physical and Mental Well-Being Throughout Life

Scientific discussions of the interplay between biological factors (nature) and environmental factors (nurture) have been going on for centuries.[25] Multiple levels of

Box 1
Grand challenge goal B: advance prevention and implementation of early interventions

Challenge 1: Support community environments that promote physical and mental well-being throughout life

Challenge 2: Develop interventions to reduce the long-term negative impact of low childhood socioeconomic status on cognitive ability and mental health

Challenge 3: Develop locally appropriate strategies to eliminate childhood abuse and enhance child protection

Challenge 4: Develop an evidence-based set of primary prevention interventions for a range of mental, neurologic, and substance use disorders

Challenge 5: Reduce the duration of untreated illness by developing culturally sensitive early interventions across settings

Adapted from Collins PY, Patel V, Joestl SS, et al. Grand challenges in global mental health. Nature 2011;475:27–30.

environmental exposures affect child development and well-being, including intrauterine exposures and the postnatal and early life influences of nutrition, infectious disease, and exposure to toxic agents.[26–28] Socioeconomic status also drives exposure to risk and protective factors that have a significant impact on children's physical, social, and cognitive development.[29–32] Neighborhoods, usually a function of socioeconomic status, matter, too. Concentrated disadvantage in wealthy countries is associated with violence, depression, and increased mortality.[33] An urban US study among 5- to 11-year-old children demonstrated increasing prevalence of mental health problems across neighborhoods with increasing levels of poverty. Collective efficacy, a neighborhood social process the researchers measured, was associated with better mental health outcomes and mediated the effects of concentrated disadvantage.[34]

Research findings such as these have the potential to inform public health policy and practice. The UK Government Office for Science sponsored a nationwide research program to examine the contextual exposures that influence well-being over the life course: the Foresight Project on Mental Capital and Wellbeing.[35,36] The project organizers convened a multidisciplinary group of investigators and policy makers in order to provide recommendations to the government on how best to achieve mental well-being, develop mental capital, and ultimately create a flourishing society in the United Kingdom over the next 20 years. They defined mental development in terms of mental capital and mental well-being. Mental capital represents cognitive and emotional resources (cognitive ability, flexibility and efficiency at learning, emotional intelligence, and social skills), and mental well-being refers to an individual's ability to develop his or her potential, work productively, and creatively build strong and positive relationships with others and contribute to the community.[35] Adopting a life course approach, the organizers outlined biological, relational, cultural, and environmental exposures across the developmental trajectory that increase the risk for poor mental and physical health outcomes and enhance mental capital and well-being. **Fig. 1** depicts these interactions over the life span. Perhaps most importantly, the project poses questions relevant to implementation—"to what extent should policy choices take account of mental capital and well-being"—and highlights existing government initiatives informed by the project's synthesis.[36]

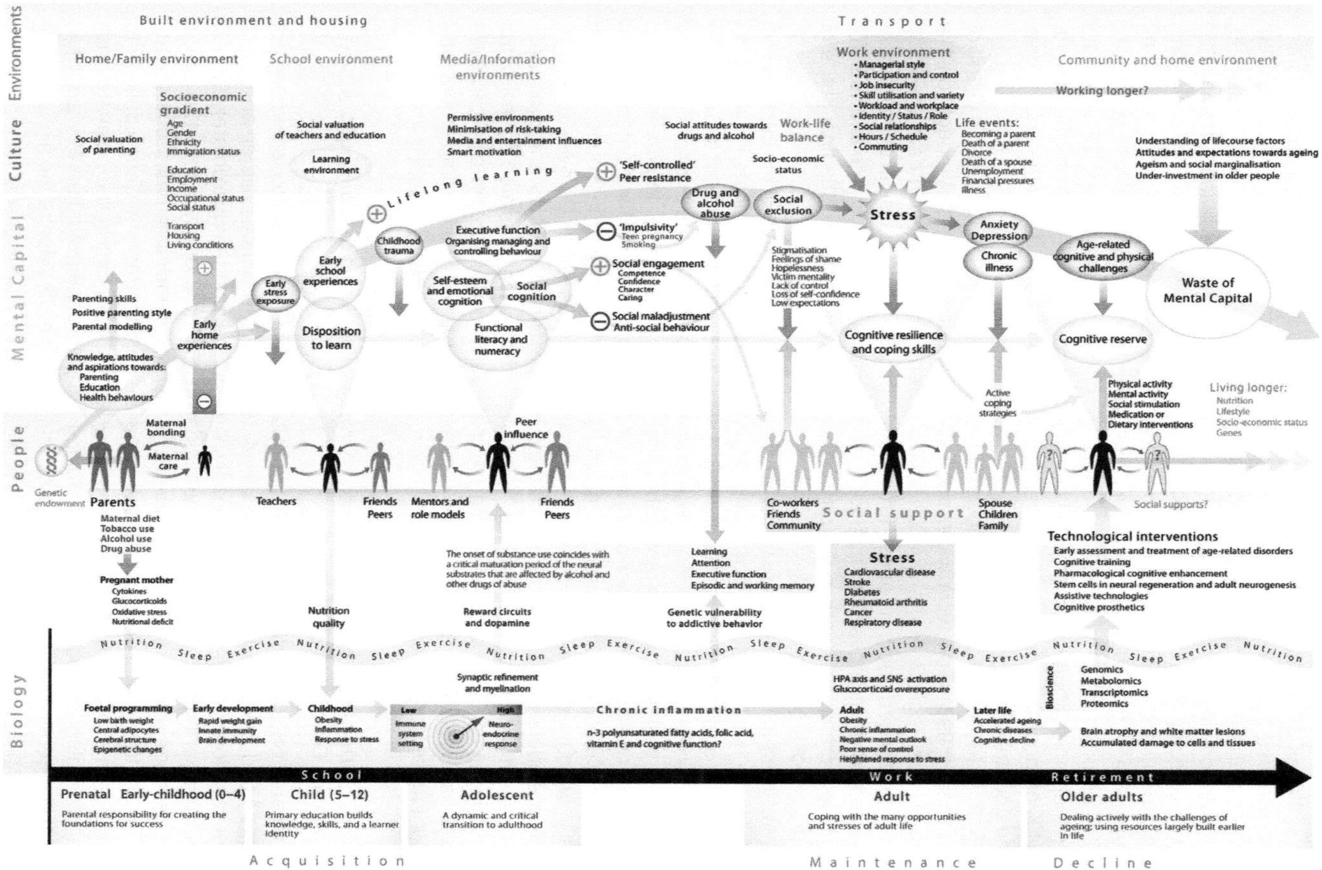

Fig. 1. Positive and negative influences on mental capital and mental well-being over the life course. (*From* Foresight Mental Capital and Wellbeing Project. Final project report: executive summary. London: The Government Office for Science; 2008. Available at: https://www.gov.uk/government/uploads/system/uploads/attachment_data/file/292453/mental-capital-wellbeing-summary.pdf.)

Challenge 2: Develop Interventions to Reduce the Long-Term Negative Impact of Low Childhood Socioeconomic Status on Cognitive Ability and Mental Health

Experiences and genes build the neural architecture of the developing brain.[12] Cognitive, emotional, physical, and social health potential emerges from the complex integrative processes of the brain as it continuously interacts with the social and environmental context.[12] Poverty is associated with reduced access to basic services, poor sanitation and associated risks for infection, and undernutrition—factors that adversely affect growth and neurodevelopment, cognition, and mental health. Not surprisingly, people living in poverty disproportionately experience mental disorders and their sequelae.[37,38] Although the number of people living in extreme poverty decreased from 1.9 billion in 1990 to 1.2 billion in 2010,[39] children younger than 13 years are among the poorest population group in developing countries.[40] These children constitute 34% of those living in extreme poverty, and they make up 50% of the poor in low-income countries.[40]

In 2012, a United Nations study showed that 1 in 7 children younger than 5 years, or approximately 99 million worldwide, were underweight for age.[39] Although on the decline in most regions of the world, 1 in 4 children in the world—an estimated 162 million—are stunted and thus at risk for impaired cognitive and physical development and related consequences such as poor school performance.[39,41] In one analysis, for every 10% increase in stunting, the proportion of children reaching the final grade of primary school dropped by 7.9%.[41]

Several international efforts are underway to use the current state of the evidence on ECD to move health systems, governments, and funders to appropriate implementation of health and social interventions. In 2013, United Nations Children's Fund published the *Handbook of Early Child Development Research and its Impact on Global Policy*, a text that synthesizes research evidence that these major threats—poverty, conflict, and disease—endanger children's chances of achieving their potential. The Institute of Medicine (IOM) launched a forum in 2014, Investing in Young Children Globally, which will convene key stakeholders from LMICs and HICs over 3 years to "translate evidence into sound and strategic investments in policies and practices" for the benefit of children and families.[42] The World Bank has translated the evidence for investing in ECD into a free e-learning format so that decision makers can educate themselves about ECD, prioritize needs for their settings, and finance, implement, and monitor intersectoral interventions.[43]

Challenge 3: Develop Locally Appropriate Strategies to Eliminate Childhood Abuse and Enhance Child Protection

An estimated 681,000 children in the United States were victims of abuse and neglect in 2011,[44] and the United States is not alone. Violence inflicted on children and youth occurs in various forms and can be deadly. Around the world, approximately 95,000 people younger than 20 years died of homicides in 2012.[45] Globally, about 120 million girls experience some form of coerced sex at least once in their lifetimes.[45] Inadequate social protections and social norms that condone some forms of violence collude to keep children at risk.[45] Child abuse has long-term effects that include elevated risk of drug and alcohol abuse, sexual risk-taking behaviors, perpetuation of violence in subsequent generations, and poor educational outcomes.[46] Despite the global nature of violence against children, only 1 prevention study from LMICs was published between 1995 and 2011.[46] The authors present examples of intervention components and study findings in **Table 1**. Effective evidence-based interventions to reduce child abuse have long existed,[47] but access to such interventions is not universal.

Table 1
Summary of selected findings for mental disorder prevention and mental health promotion interventions

Intervention Category	Intervention Components	Exemplary Outcome Measures (List)	Global Distribution of Research (Yes or No)	Main Findings	Research Gaps
Child abuse prevention	ECHV (provide support, education, improve child health & caregiving) PE (provide education, improve child-rearing skills) School-based CSA programs (education) MCT (family support, parenting skills, preschool education)	Child maltreatment (hospital visits, parental report, referrals to protective services) Parenting skills Parental employment & reliance on social services	No 0.6% of research from LMICs Reviewed in Skeen and Tomlinson,[46] 2013 and Mikton and Butchart,[89] 2009	ECHV: reduced risk factors for child maltreatment Only clear evidence of reduced actual maltreatment: Nurse-family partnership (USA) PE: some small to medium effects for reduction in risk factors and actual maltreatment, others only on reduced risk factors CSA: mixed—increased knowledge, no clear evidence of reduced abuse MCT: moderate effects in some studies, mixed evidence regarding reduction of risk factors in others	Improve methodological quality in HIC studies (use of control groups, internal validity, randomized controlled designs) Overall prevention interventions in LMICs
Early childhood education	Parent training: 1. Improving parenting practices (eg, increased sensitive responsive interactions and early stimulation) 2. Emotional support for parents Center based: 1. Training teachers/caregivers in behavior management and greater social, emotional, and coping skills	Observation of child behavior Assessment of child attachment Assessment of child mental health Assessment of caregiver practices (eg, measures of parenting) Assessment of caregiver mental health	Yes Reviewed in Baker-Henningham,[90] 2014	Overall improvements in child mental health outcomes, and behavioral outcomes (both in short term [12/16 studies] and long term [6/6 studies]) Benefits in caregiver practices (21/25 studies) and caregiver mental health (6/9 studies)	Need more long-term follow-up studies Discern optimal timing and duration Assess benefit to other children in the family Effect of booster interventions during later part of childhood

(*continued on next page*)

Table 1
(continued)

Intervention Category	Intervention Components	Exemplary Outcome Measures (List)	Global Distribution of Research (Yes or No)	Main Findings	Research Gaps
Mental health promotion interventions	Cognitive behavioral frameworks to structure building socioemotional skills, problem solving, and increased positive behaviors Physical, reproductive, and psychological health education Stress reduction techniques	Emotional and behavioral well-being (eg, self-esteem, self-efficacy, coping skills, prosocial behaviors) Mental health assessment (anxiety, depression, PTSD, anger, hyperactivity symptoms)	Yes Reviewed in Barry et al,[70] 2013	Positive effects for children living in conflict areas Mixed results in other interventions with differential gender and age group effects Positive effects in life skill and resilience-building programs	Discern optimal components of intervention (age, individual/group, timing, duration) Need more research in low-income countries and in younger age groups (5–10 y) Assess cost-effectiveness
School-based mental health interventions	Health promotion: see mental health promotion intervention components and outcome measures described above Prevention and treatment (can be universal, selective and indicated): Cognitive behavioral techniques Creative arts and relaxation techniques Multimodal (including family and community components)	Health promotion: see mental health promotion intervention components and outcomes described above Prevention and treatment: mental health assessment (anxiety, depression, PTSD, anger, hyperactivity symptoms)	Yes Reviewed in Barry et al,[70] 2013 and Fazel et al,[69] 2014	In LMICs: most positive effects on PTSD symptoms Mixed effects on depression, grief, behaviors, and conduct symptoms Differential sex effects as well as differential effects depending on symptom severity	Discern optimal components of intervention Develop outcome measures that integrate mental health and academic outcomes Assessment fidelity of interventions Need more long-term follow-up studies

Early intervention for psychosis	Prodromal symptoms: CBT Specialized team[a] Medications Omega-3 fatty acids Transition to psychosis: CBT vs supportive counseling Omega-3 fatty acids Improving outcome of first-episode psychosis: Medications CBT Family therapy Specialized team Vocational training	Transition to psychosis Adherence to treatment Number of hospitalizations and number of days hospitalized Living independently Working or studying	No (1 study in China, the rest in HICs) Reviewed in Marshal and Rathbone,[92] 2011; Stafford et al,[93] 2013	Prodromal symptoms: No effects of antipsychotics or CBT alone. Short-term effects of combination of all 3 over specialized team alone. Not sustained at 1 year Possible benefit of Omega-3 fatty acids Reduced transition to psychosis: Moderate-quality evidence in favor of CBT vs supportive counseling Low-quality evidence in favor of omega-3 fatty acids vs placebo Improving outcome of first-episode psychosis: Some support for vocational training and family therapy in addition to medications	Rigorous randomized controlled trials Studies in LMICs Improved characterization of the role of a specialized team and the intervention components

Abbreviations: CBT, cognitive behavioral therapy; CSA, child sexual abuse; ECHV, early childhood home visitation; MCT, multicomponent; PE, parent education; PTSD, posttraumatic stress disorder.

[a] Specialized team is a multidisciplinary psychiatric team specializing in the treatment of patients with first-episode psychosis.

Data from Refs.[46,69,70,89–93]

In response to these challenges, the United States Agency for International Development convened an Evidence Summit in 2011 to assess the available research that could inform strategies for policies and programs supporting child protection in LMIC. The Action Plan on Children in Adversity emerged from this process as a means of integrating sound practices into development initiatives.[48] The plan uses existing evidence to promote strategies that support child development, prevent family separation, and promote safe and permanent family care, and to protect children from violence and abuse. The implementation of the plan calls for interagency collaboration within the US government as well as in the collaborating countries, which will aim to achieve progress toward these goals by 2017. At the same time, the US Centers for Disease Control and Prevention's Violence Against Children Survey permits countries supported by the President's Emergency Plan for AIDS Relief (PEPFAR) to measure the prevalence of violence as a first step toward applying remedies.

Challenge 4: Develop an Evidence-Based Set of Primary Prevention Interventions for a Range of Mental, Neurologic, and Substance Use Disorders

Understanding the multiple causes of mental disorders and developing effective interventions to prevent them remain grand challenges. Existing prevention interventions typically focus on a specific disorder and can be classified as universal (targeting the entire eligible population), selective (targeting a population at risk for illness), or indicated (targeting a population with subthreshold symptoms of disease).[49] The IOM and National Research Council's 2009 report, *Preventing Mental, Emotional and Behavioral Disorders in Young People*, synthesizes the evidence for prevention and encourages an expanded focus that moves beyond preventing illness to include promoting wellness, collaborating between neuroscience and prevention science, using an interagency approach, being responsive to community priorities, focusing on dissemination and implementation research, including cost analyses, and concurrent screening and intervention activities.[50]

Although sometimes overshadowed by treatment-focused research, the global evidence base for preventive interventions for mental disorders is varied and expanding.[15,51–53] Most intervention studies come from HICs and are disease focused, targeting common mental disorders in childhood such as depression,[54–56] anxiety,[57–60] conduct disorder,[61–64] and substance abuse.[65–68] A few of these are universal, whereas the majority have been conducted in high-risk populations. The settings for the interventions range from schools/preschools, homes, and clinics and are delivered by a range of providers: teachers, clinicians, parents, and community leaders. The duration of the interventions vary, as do the delivery (individual vs group) and the intervention content. Many use cognitive behavioral frameworks, social skills training, and parent training. Some interventions target youth directly, and others focus on parents and primary caregivers. Recent systematic reviews on the effectiveness of mental health promotion interventions in youth in LMICs found good evidence for the effectiveness of selected interventions to reduce anxiety and depressive symptoms and enhance self-esteem, self-efficacy, and motivation in youth[69,70] (see **Table 1**). Schools emerged as an important context for interventions focused on children affected by conflict, but a sizable number of interventions had no effect.

Although more research is needed to clarify targets for preventive interventions, existing effective interventions merit attention for scaling up. One of the 4 objectives of the WHO Comprehensive Mental Health Action Plan 2013–2020 is to "implement strategies for prevention and promotion in mental health." The World Health Assembly adopted the plan in 2013, and the plan, with its accompanying resolution, was an assertion of commitment from WHO's 194 member states to achieve the plan's objectives.[71]

Challenge 5: Reduce the Duration of Untreated Illness by Developing Culturally Sensitive Early Interventions Across Settings

Psychotic disorders may be among the most widely recognized mental illnesses worldwide, and they frequently begin in adolescence. A significant body of mental health research on the duration of untreated illness focuses on these disorders. Data from HICs suggest, however, that psychotic symptoms, per se, are not uncommon, occurring in 4% to 8% of the general population, and the prevalence may be higher among children and adolescents.[72] A community study of youth aged 14 to 29 years from Kenya reported that 45% of the sample endorsed at least 1 psychotic risk symptom.[73] These experiences do not necessarily predict the onset of a psychotic disorder; rather, they are apt to be indicators of risk for a variety of mental disorders (including depression, bipolar disorder, and sometimes schizophrenia). Even when psychotic symptoms do represent a prodrome for psychotic disorders (usually schizophrenia spectrum disorders), approximately 18% to 36% of people defined as high risk go on to transition to a mental disorder, with the risk of transition increasing over time.[72] Once the transition occurs, a minority of patients achieve recovery, and a longer duration of untreated psychosis (DUP) is associated with greater morbidity. Identifying who is at risk to transition to a psychotic disorder, and intervening early, remains a critical area for investigation. Efforts to harmonize data across research sites in HICs enrich these research activities, but questions remain about the validity of commonly used measures to assess those who may be at high risk for psychosis in low-income country settings[73] (see **Table 1**).

Among those who do develop a psychotic disorder, the DUP is associated with more severe symptoms, decreased remission rates, poor social functioning, and poorer overall functioning and quality of life among individuals in HIC and LMIC.[74–76] The mean duration of untreated illness differs significantly between HICs and LMICs with almost double the duration in the latter.[77] A recent UK study showed higher DUP among adolescents, and within that group, Asians had the lowest DUP, followed by black participants, and then white adolescents.[78] Studies in Indonesia[79] and China[80] have reported increased mortality associated with prolonged duration of untreated illness. In these examples, the lack of available mental health services likely contributes to the chronicity and morbidity associated with psychotic disorders. The WHO Comprehensive Mental Health Action Plan 2013–2020 identifies a 20% increase in service coverage for severe mental disorders by 2020 as a target,[5] but identifying and integrating evidence-based interventions for the prevention of psychosis into these services will require additional research.

BUILDING RESEARCH CAPACITY

Meeting the grand challenges relevant to CAMH requires a skilled global, collaborative, multidisciplinary research workforce with the capacity to translate research findings to practice settings in health, education, and other relevant sectors. Although several training programs in global mental health have emerged over the past 5 years, developing and sustaining a global cadre of CAMH researchers will require that several interacting factors be addressed.[18] Countries must provide training and capacity-building opportunities for the development of skills in the basic, translational, and implementation sciences; the necessary research infrastructure; adequate financial resources; and environments that facilitate the conduct of research in order to address research priorities.[18] In LMICs, the dearth of mental health clinical providers contributes to limited mental health research activity, as do the lack of graduate programs and the pressing need for clinical service providers to devote their energies to patient care.[81]

Other barriers curtail traditional research career trajectories. Once trained, new researchers must be mentored and retained. In LMICs, clinical and teaching responsibilities limit the available time to conduct research and clinical faculty seldom receive salaries to conduct research.[18] The brain drain, that is, the loss of an already limited skilled workforce to higher resourced organizations or countries, demands innovative retention efforts. When trainees from LMICs receive research training in HICs, sufficient infrastructure must exist in the home institution in order to make returning worthwhile. Initiatives such as the Medical Education Partnership Initiative (MEPI), funded by the US National Institutes of Health and the President's Emergency Plan for AIDS Relief (PEPFAR), address some of these concerns. MEPI aims to enhance medical education so that health systems function effectively to deliver services in countries supported by PEPFAR. The initiative's specific aims are to build clinical capacity, retain clinicians, and stimulate and support contextually relevant research by building research capacity.[82] MEPI provides funds to extend and reform clinical training approaches in 12 African countries, while also exposing students and trainees to research opportunities.[82]

MEPI programs in Kenya and Zimbabwe provide mental health research training opportunities, specifically linked to larger medical education efforts. The University of Zimbabwe's initiative, Improving Mental Health Education and Research capacity in Zimbabwe offered scholarships to develop new academic psychiatrists, master classes taught by international experts in child psychiatry and other underrepresented areas of training, and research training and mentoring opportunities.[83] Among the lessons learned, the team noted the importance of building clinical service training and research experiences around needs in the local context. Mentorship by external experts was valued and best accomplished through teamwork and skills transfer in person with continuity through electronic communications. The program experienced a 4-fold increase in psychiatry faculty over 4 years and witnessed growth in its postgraduate training program.

Mentorship plays an important role in faculty development and success in every setting. Mentors guide trainees or junior faculty to resources and model skills not formally taught (eg, time management, perseverance).[18] Mentors provide the "roadmap of a research career and help to correct naïve assumptions" and assist with informed decision making about alternate career paths.[18,84] Here again, the limited number of researchers in mental health, globally, also limits the number of available mentors. The challenge of finding a mentor is not restricted to LMICs; early career researchers in North America also face the small number of North American researchers focused on global mental health themes. Existing faculty must carve out time for mentorship amid competing priorities. In both high-income and low-income settings, up and coming researchers can experience isolation because of the dearth of investigators with shared or overlapping interests.[18]

Are there incentives for mentorship in LMIC academic institutions? Many of these institutions face challenges analogous to those faced by non–research-intensive institutions in the United States, where heavy teaching or administrative responsibilities compete with opportunities for research. Collins and colleagues[18] note that in institutions without a culture of research or a strong research infrastructure, the senior faculty expected to mentor students and the junior faculty may not have received adequate training in research methods and grant writing or may not have strong publication records. Partnering with research-intensive institutions or experienced teams can help solve this problem. The National Institute of Mental Health-supported Collaborative Hubs for International Research on Mental Health provide one such example (http://www.nimh.nih.gov/about/organization/od/globalhubs/index.shtml). These 5 collaborative research teams conduct research aimed at reducing the mental health treatment gap in LMICs. Each funded hub consists of collaborating teams from 4 or more countries in a given region; they serve as regional resources for research training opportunities that occur through short courses, research mentorship, and on-the-job training for research assistants and coordinators.

Research partnerships also provide opportunities for researchers to develop skills for equitable collaboration. In the context of collaboration, teams confront the realities of differential resource distribution in the form of salaries, expertise, access to funding, and research human resources. How will these differences influence relationships across teams? How will pressures related to career maintenance, funding acquisition, advancement, and promotion among HIC investigators influence decision making? Will collaborations result in the development of new research leaders among the teams with fewer resources? Such teams are more frequently represented among LMIC organizations or institutions in HICs that are less research intensive.

Researchers working across cultural and economic contexts also confront the need for careful attention to ethical research practices. Research with children and other vulnerable populations—often made more vulnerable in the context of poverty—requires oversight by ethics committees or institutional review boards. As researchers obtain informed consent for research participation, they will need to understand and be sensitive to decision-making processes in the local context and meanings of privacy and confidentiality.[85] Ruiz-Casares[85] recommends that research teams "create safe spaces for reflection and dialogue on the scientific and ethical principles relevant to mental health research and the cultural, social, and other factors that may facilitate or hinder the conditions under study."

Skills for ethical and equitable collaboration can also be operationalized through learning to prepare and disseminate research findings. Kohrt and colleagues[86] outline procedures for collaborative writing that results in equitable representation of collaborators from LMICs on academic publications. The investigators observe that a key component involves "distributing lead authorship for different outputs at the same time as having mechanisms in place (eg, mentoring, workshops, coursework) to develop skills needed to adequately perform the role of lead author."

In addition to writing skills for academic publications, global mental health research teams can benefit from learning to translate and disseminate research findings to local stakeholders and decision makers. The diversity of member roles on collaborative research teams, which likely include clinicians and other practitioners (eg, teachers, peers, lay health workers) as well as other community members, is a distinct advantage. Building research capacity affords opportunities to train nontraditional researchers in research methods. Teams can craft research training as a route to educate mental health service users. Teams can also train health system decision makers on the applications of research to meet public health needs. Initiatives like the Mental Health Leadership and Advocacy Program in West Africa do precisely this.[87] The project teaches mental health care providers, government officials, policymakers, and organizations representing service users and caregivers about mental health and builds skills for advocating for mental health service development among key stakeholders.[87] The leaders that emerge from such programs are ideal candidates for research training. Although they may not conduct research, understanding the sources and uses of local data can further empower them.

SUMMARY

The 5 challenges discussed here demand more than multidisciplinary research efforts. These challenges require coordinated efforts across science, policy, and many domains of practice (education, nutrition, mental health, justice, etc.). The authors have described specific programs that attempt to mobilize the diverse skills of multiple stakeholders to tackle these problems. Can a larger effort be mounted? The global effort to expand access to treatment and care for human immunodeficiency virus infection is a good example of a public health effort that garnered large, targeted investments and rapidly linked new evidence to clinical practice, making use of partnerships among funders, governments, scientists, clinicians, advocates, and community organizations.[88] There are surely lessons for mental health researchers and other interested parties. The stakes are high: they carry the life chances of millions of children worldwide for whom research is critical and the capacity to move relevant research to action, essential.

REFERENCES

1. WHO. Preventing suicide: a global perspective. Geneva (Switzerland): World Health Organization; 2014.
2. WHO. Health for the World's adolescents: a second chance in the second decade, summary. Geneva (Switzerland): World Health Organization; 2014.
3. Herne MA, Bartholomew ML, Weahkee RL. Suicide mortality among American Indians and Alaska natives, 1999-2009. Am J Public Health 2014;104:S336–42.
4. Hicks J. Statistical data on death by suicide by Nunavut Inuit, 1920 to 2014. Report prepared for Nunavut Tunngavik Inc; 2015.
5. WHO. Mental health action plan 2013-2020. Geneva (Switzerland): World Health Organization; 2013.
6. National Action Alliance for Suicide Prevention. Research prioritization task force. a prioritized research agenda for suicide prevention: an action plan to save lives. Rockville (MD): National Institute of Mental Health and the Research Prioritization Task Force; 2014.
7. United Nations Department of Economic and Social Affairs, Population Division. World population prospects: the 2012 revision. DVD Edition. New York: United Nations; 2013.
8. Kessler RC, Amminger GP, Aguilar-Gaxiola S, et al. Age of onset of mental disorders: a review of recent literature. Curr Opin Psychiatry 2007;20:359–64.
9. Kessler RC, Berglund P, Demler O, et al. Lifetime prevalence and age-of-onset distributions of DSM-IV disorders in the National Comorbidity Survey Replication. Arch Gen Psychiatry 2005;62:593–602.
10. Murray C, Vos T, Lozano R, et al. Disability-adjusted life years (DALYs) for 291 diseases and injuries in 21 regions, 1990-2010: a systematic analysis for the Global Burden of Disease Study 2010. Lancet 2012;380:2197–223.
11. Vos T, Flaxman A, Naghavi M, et al. Years lived with disability (YLDs) for 1160 sequelae of 289 diseases and injuries 1990-2010: a systematic analysis for the Global Burden of Disease Study 2010. Lancet 2012;380:2163–96.
12. Shonkoff JP, Richter L. The powerful reach of early childhood development: a science-based foundation for sound investment. In: Britto PR, Engle PL, Super CM, editors. Handbook of early childhood development research and its impact on global policy. New York: Oxford University Press; 2013. p. 24–34.
13. Insel TR. Mental disorders in childhood: shifting the focus from behavioral symptoms to neurodevelopmental trajectories. JAMA 2014;311:1727–8.

14. Commission on Health Research for Development. Health Research: essential link to equity in development. New York: Oxford University Press; 1990.
15. Kieling C, Baker-Henningham H, Belfer M, et al. Child and adolescent mental health worldwide: evidence for action. Lancet 2011;378:1515–25.
16. Hoagwood K, Olin S. The NIMH blueprint for change report: research priorities in child and adolescent mental health. J Am Acad Child Adolesc Psychiatry 2002; 41:760–7.
17. Moon S, Szlezák NA, Michaud CM, et al. The global health system: lessons for a stronger institutional framework. PLoS Med 2010;7:e1000193.
18. Collins PY, Tomlinson M, Kakuma R, et al. Research priorities, capacity, and networks in global mental health. In: Patel V, Minas H, Cohen A, et al, editors. Global mental health principles and practice. New York: Oxford University Press; 2013. p. 425–49.
19. Varmus H, Klausner R, Zerhouni E, et al. Grand challenges in global health. Science 2003;302:398–9.
20. Daar AS, Singer PA, Persad DL, et al. Grand challenges in chronic non-communicable diseases. Nature 2007;450:494–6.
21. Collins PY, Patel V, Joestl SS, et al. Grand challenges in global mental health. Nature 2011;475:27–30.
22. Lancet Mental Health Group, Chisholm D, Flisher AJ, et al. Scale up services for mental disorders: a call for action. Lancet 2007;370:1241–52.
23. Sharan P, Gallo C, Gureje O, et al. Mental health research priorities in low- and middle-income countries of Africa, Asia, Latin America and the Caribbean. Br J Psychiatry 2009;195:354–63.
24. Tomlinson M, Rudan I, Saxena S, et al. Setting priorities for global mental health research. Bull World Health Organ 2009;87:438–46.
25. Galton F. English men of science: their nature and nurture. London: Macmillan & co; 1874.
26. Rees S, Harding R. Brain development during fetal life: influences of the intra-uterine environment. Neurosci Lett 2004;361:111–4.
27. Irner TB, Teasdale TW, Olofsson M. Cognitive and social development in preschool children born to women using substances. J Addict Dis 2012;31:29–44.
28. Perera FP, Rauh V, Whyatt RM, et al. A summary of recent findings on birth outcomes and developmental effects of prenatal ETS, PAH, and pesticide exposures. Neurotoxicology 2005;26:573–87.
29. Bradley RH, Corwyn RF. Socioeconomic status and child development. Annu Rev Psychol 2002;53:371–99.
30. Hackman DA, Farah MJ, Meaney MJ. Socioeconomic status and the brain: mechanistic insights from human and animal research. Nat Rev Neurosci 2010;11: 651–9.
31. Walker SP, Wachs TD, Gardner JM, et al. Child development: risk factors for adverse outcomes in developing countries. Lancet 2007;369:145–57.
32. Berkman DS, Lescano AG, Gilman RH, et al. Effects of stunting, diarrhoeal disease, and parasitic infection during infancy on cognition in late childhood: a follow-up study. Lancet 2002;359:564–71.
33. Sampson RJ. The neighborhood context of well-being. Perspect Biol Med 2003; 46:S53–64.
34. Xue Y, Leventhal T, Brooks-Gunn J, et al. Neighborhood residence and mental health problems of 5- to 11-year-olds. Arch Gen Psychiatry 2005;62:554–63.
35. Beddington J, Cooper CL, Field J, et al. The mental wealth of nations. Nature 2008;455:1057–60.

36. Foresight mental capital and wellbeing project. Final project report. London: The Government Office for Science; 2008.
37. Patel V, Kleinman A. Poverty and common mental disorders in developing countries. Bull World Health Organ 2003;81:609–15.
38. Lund C, De Silva M, Plagerson S, et al. Poverty and mental disorders: breaking the cycle in low-income and middle-income countries. Lancet 2011;378:1502–14.
39. United Nations. The millennium development goals report. New York: United Nations; 2014.
40. Olinto P, Beegle K, Sobrado C, et al. The state of the poor: Where are the poor, where is extreme poverty harder to end, and what is the current profile of the world's poor? Economic Premise 2013. Available at: http://www.worldbank.org/economicpremise. Accessed November 22, 2014.
41. Grantham-McGregor S, Cheung YB, Cueto S, et al. Developmental potential in the first 5 years for children in developing countries. Lancet 2007;369:60–70.
42. IOM (Institute of Medicine), National Research Council. The cost of inaction for young children globally: workshop summary. Washington, DC: National Academies Press; 2014.
43. The World Bank. Education Staff Development Program: Early Childhood Development for Policymakers and Practitioners. 2014. Available at: http://einstitute.worldbank.org/ei/course/education-staff-development-program-early-childhood-development-policymakers-and-practitioner. Accessed November 22, 2014.
44. U.S. Department of Health and Human Services, Administration for Children and Families, Administration on Children Youth and Families, Children's Bureau, Child Maltreatment 2011. 2012. Available at: http://www.acf.hhs.gov/programs/cb/research-data-technology/statistics-research/child-maltreatment. Accessed November 22, 2014.
45. United Nations Children's Fund. Hidden in Plain Sight: a statistical analysis of violence against children. New York: UNICEF; 2014.
46. Skeen S, Tomlinson M. A public health approach to preventing child abuse in low- and middle-income countries: a call for action. Int J Psychol 2013;48:108–16.
47. Olds DL, Henderson J, Charles R, et al. Preventing child abuse and neglect: a randomized trial of nurse home visitation. Pediatrics 1986;78:65–78.
48. USAID. United States Government Action Plan on Children In Adversity: A Framework for International Assistance: 2012-2017. 2012. Available at: http://www.usaid.gov/sites/default/files/documents/1860/United States Action Plan on Children in Adversity.pdf. Accessed November 22, 2014.
49. Gordon RS Jr. An operational classification of disease prevention. Public Health Rep 1983;98:107–9.
50. Institute of Medicine, National Research Council. Preventing mental, emotional, and behavioral disorders among young people: progress and possibilities. Washington, DC: The National Academies Press; 2009.
51. Jane-Llopis E, Barry M, Hosman C, et al. Mental health promotion works: a review. Promot Educ 2005;(Suppl 2):9–25, 61, 67.
52. World Health Organization. Promoting mental health: concepts, emerging evidence, practice: summary report/a report from the World Health Organization, Department of Mental Health and Substance Abuse in collaboration with the Victorian Health Promotion Foundation and the University of Melbourne. Geneva, Switzerland: World Health Organization; 2004.
53. Hosman C, Lopis J. Political challenges 2: Mental health. The Evidence of Health Promotion Effectiveness: Shaping Public Health in a New Europe. International

Union for Health Promotion and Education, IUHPE. Paris: Jouve Composition & Impression; 1999. p. 29–41.
54. Brunwasser SM, Gillham JE, Kim ES. A meta-analytic review of the Penn Resiliency Program's effect on depressive symptoms. J Consult Clin Psychol 2009; 77:1042–54.
55. Clarke GN, Hawkins W, Murphy M, et al. Targeted prevention of unipolar depressive disorder in an at-risk sample of high school adolescents: a randomized trial of a group cognitive intervention. J Am Acad Child Adolesc Psychiatry 1995;34:312–21.
56. Arnarson EÖ, Craighead WE. Prevention of depression among Icelandic adolescents. Behav Res Ther 2009;47:577–85.
57. Barrett PM, Farrell LJ, Ollendick TH, et al. Long-term outcomes of an Australian universal prevention trial of anxiety and depression symptoms in children and youth: an evaluation of the friends program. J Clin Child Adolesc Psychol 2006; 35:403–11.
58. Dadds MR, Roth JH. Prevention of anxiety disorders: results of a universal trial with young children. J Child Fam Stud 2008;17:320–35.
59. Stallard P. Mental health prevention in UK classrooms: the FRIENDS anxiety prevention programme. Emot Behav Diffic 2010;15:23–35.
60. Lowry-Webster HM, Barrett PM, Dadds MR. A universal prevention trial of anxiety and depressive symptomatology in childhood: preliminary data from an Australian study. Behav Change 2001;18:36–50.
61. Webster-Stratton C, Jamila Reid M, Stoolmiller M. Preventing conduct problems and improving school readiness: evaluation of the incredible years teacher and child training programs in high-risk schools. J Child Psychol Psychiatry 2008; 49:471–88.
62. Slough NM, McMahon RJ, Bierman KL, et al. Preventing Serious conduct problems in school-age youths: the fast track program. Cogn Behav Pract 2008;15:3–17.
63. McCord J, Tremblay RE, Vitaro F, et al. Boys' disruptive behaviour, school adjustment, and delinquency: the Montreal prevention experiment. Int J Behav Dev 1994;17:739–52.
64. Ialongo N, Poduska J, Werthamer L, et al. The distal impact of two first-grade preventive interventions on conduct problems and disorder in early adolescence. J Emot Behav Disord 2001;9:146–60.
65. Palinkas LA, Atkins CJ, Miller C, et al. Social skills training for drug prevention in high-risk female adolescents. Prev Med 1996;25:692–701.
66. Griffin KW, Botvin GJ, Nichols TR, et al. Effectiveness of a universal drug abuse prevention approach for youth at high risk for substance use initiation. Prev Med 2003;36:1–7.
67. Pantin H, Prado G, Lopez B, et al. A randomized controlled trial of Familias Unidas for Hispanic adolescents with behavior problems. Psychosom Med 2009;71: 987–95.
68. Conrod PJ, Castellanos-Ryan N, Strang J. Brief, personality-targeted coping skills interventions and survival as a non-drug user over a 2-year period during adolescence. Arch Gen Psychiatry 2010;67:85–93.
69. Fazel M, Patel V, Thomas S, et al. Mental health interventions in schools in low-income and middle-income countries. Lancet Psychiatry 2014;1:388–98.
70. Barry MM, Clarke AM, Jenkins R, et al. A systematic review of the effectiveness of mental health promotion interventions for young people in low and middle income countries. BMC Public Health 2013;13:835.
71. Saxena S, Funk M, Chisholm D. World health assembly adopts comprehensive mental health action plan 2013–2020. Lancet 2013;381:1970–1.

72. Fusar-Poli P, Borgwardt S, Bechdolf A, et al. The psychosis high-risk state: a comprehensive state-of-the-art review. JAMA Psychiatry 2013;70:107–20.
73. Mamah D, Mbwayo A, Mutiso V, et al. A survey of psychosis risk symptoms in Kenya. Compr Psychiatry 2012;53:516–24.
74. Penttila M, Jaaskelainen E, Hirvonen N, et al. Duration of untreated psychosis as predictor of long-term outcome in schizophrenia: systematic review and meta-analysis. Br J Psychiatry 2014;205:88–94.
75. Marshall M, Lewis S, Lockwood A, et al. Association between duration of untreated psychosis and outcome in cohorts of first-episode patients: a systematic review. Arch Gen Psychiatry 2005;62:975–83.
76. Farooq S, Large M, Nielssen O, et al. The relationship between the duration of untreated psychosis and outcome in low-and-middle income countries: a systematic review and meta analysis. Schizophr Res 2009;109:15–23.
77. Large M, Farooq S, Nielssen O, et al. Relationship between gross domestic product and duration of untreated psychosis in low- and middle-income countries. Br J Psychiatry 2008;193:272–8.
78. Fraguas D, Merchán-Naranjo J, del Rey-Mejías Á, et al. A longitudinal study on the relationship between duration of untreated psychosis and executive function in early-onset first-episode psychosis. Schizophr Res 2014;158:126–33.
79. Kurihara T, Kato M, Kashima H, et al. Excess mortality of schizophrenia in the developing country of Bali. Schizophr Res 2006;83:103–5.
80. Ran MS, Chen EY, Conwell Y, et al. Mortality in people with schizophrenia in rural China: 10-year cohort study. Br J Psychiatry 2007;190:237–42.
81. Thornicroft G, Cooper S, Bortel TV, et al. Capacity building in global mental health research. Harv Rev Psychiatry 2012;20:13–24.
82. Mullan F, Frehywot S, Omaswa F, et al. The Medical Education Partnership Initiative: PEPFAR's effort to boost health worker education to strengthen health systems. Health Aff 2012;31:1561–72.
83. Mangezi WO, Nhiwatiwa SM, Cowan FM, et al. Improving psychiatric education and research capacity in Zimbabwe. Med Educ 2014;48:1132.
84. The Royal Society. Knowledge, networks and nations: global scientific collaboration in the 21st century. London: The Royal Society; 2011.
85. Ruiz-Casares M. Research ethics in global mental health: advancing culturally responsive mental health research. Transcult Psychiatry 2014;51:790–805.
86. Kohrt BA, Upadhaya N, Luitel NP, et al. Authorship in global mental health research: recommendations for collaborative approaches to writing and publishing. Ann Glob Health 2014;80:134–42.
87. Adbdulmalik J, Fadahunsi W, Kola L, et al. The Mental Health Leadership and Advocacy Program (mhLAP): a pioneering response to the neglect of mental health in Anglophone West Africa. Int J Ment Health Syst 2014;8:5. Available at: http://www.ijmhs.com/content/8/1/5.
88. De Cock K, El-Sadr W, Ghebreyesus T. Game changers: why did the scale-up of HIV treatment work despite weak health systems? J Acquir Immune Defic Syndr 2011;57:S61–3.
89. Mikton C, Butchart A. Child maltreatment prevention: a systematic review of reviews. Bull World Health Organ 2009;87:353–61.
90. Baker-Henningham H. The role of early childhood education programmes in the promotion of child and adolescent mental health in low- and middle-income countries. Int J Epidemiol 2014;43:407–33.
91. Fazel M, Hoagwood K, Stephan S, et al. Mental health interventions in schools in high-income countries. Lancet Psychiatry 2014;1:377–87.

92. Marshall M, Rathbone J. Early intervention for psychosis. Cochrane Database Syst Rev 2011;(6):CD004718.
93. Stafford MR, Jackson H, Mayo-Wilson E, et al. Early interventions to prevent psychosis: systematic review and meta-analysis. Br Med J 2013;346:f185.

Child and Adolescent Psychiatry Training

A Global Perspective

Ayesha I. Mian, MD[a,*], Gordana Milavić, MD, FRCPSYCH[b],
Norbert Skokauskas, MD, PhD[c]

KEYWORDS

• Training • Child and adolescent psychiatry • Children • Global • Medical education

KEY POINTS

- Different traditions and cultural contexts occasioned the development and maintenance of theoretic models and practice of child and adolescent psychiatry (CAP) depending on the teaching at the time and the influences exerted by the leaders in the profession.
- With ever-closer links at all levels across Europe and the United States, the last couple of decades have seen a quest for the standardization of teaching and training, all in the interests of children and young people and their families and the profession.
- The CAP psychiatrist will possess integrity and probity and promote health values through research and teaching.
- Child psychiatry training programs not only offer training in teaching the clinical skills of the discipline of child and adolescent psychiatry but also strive to help with the development of professionalism, ethical behaviors, and leadership skills in their trainees.

Although child and adolescent psychiatry (CAP) has now been firmly established in academic medicine for more than 50 years, the demand for child and adolescent psychiatrists continues to far outstrip the supply worldwide. There is also a severe maldistribution of child and adolescent psychiatrists, especially in rural and poor, urban areas where access is significantly reduced. Because of the concerning dearth of child and adolescent psychiatrists, and child and adolescent behavioral health providers in other disciplines, organized child psychiatry and international organizations are not only focusing on traditional training of specialists but also on innovative training

Disclosures: None.
[a] Department of Psychiatry, The Aga Khan University, National Stadium Road, Karachi 74800, Pakistan; [b] National and Specialist Services, Michael Rutter Centre, Maudsley Hospital, De'Crespigny Park, London SE5 8AZ, UK; [c] Child and Adolescent Psychiatry, Centre for Child and Adolescents Mental Health and Child Protection, Faculty of Medicine, Norwegian University of Science and Technology (NTNU), Klostergata 46, Trondheim N-7491, Norway
* Corresponding author.
E-mail address: ayesha.mian@aku.edu

programs to build capacity of health personnel at different levels of medical training as well as in other fields. This article outlines existing CAP training programs in different parts of the world and how they seek to address the growing need for trained CAP mental health personnel.

HISTORY

CAP, a relatively newer field in medicine, was not established as a specialty until the early 1900s. Early recognition of the field began in Germany, when Johannes Trüper founded a school in Sophienhöhe close to Jena, a university town, in 1892, where several physicians would gain training in child psychiatry. He was also a cofounder of *Die Kinderfehler* (1896), one of the leading journals for research in pedagogy and child psychiatry at the time. The psychiatrist and philosopher Theodor Ziehen, regarded as one of the pioneers of child psychiatry, gained practical child psychiatric experience as a consultant liaison psychiatrist at this school founded by Johannes Trüper. Around the same time in 1910, Wilhelm Strohmayer, another psychiatrist from Jena, Germany published his book *Vorlesungen uber die Psychopathologie des Kindesalters für Mediziner und Pädagogen* based on his consulting work in Sophienhöhe.[1] The discipline of CAP also regards Hermann Emminghaus as one of those responsible for it becoming established as a separate branch of science. The monograph by Emminghaus entitled "Die psychischen Störungen des Kindesalters" (Mental Disorders of Childhood), which appeared in 1887 in the *Handbuch der Kinderkrankheiten*, was the first overview in German of the emotional problems occurring during this phase of life.[2]

In 1933, Moritz Tramer, a Swiss psychiatrist, was probably the first to define the parameters of child psychiatry in terms of diagnosis, treatment, and prognosis within the discipline of medicine. In 1934, Tramer founded the *Zeitschrift für Kinderpsychiatrie (Journal of Child Psychiatry)*, which later became *Acta Paedopsychiatria.*[3] The first academic child psychiatry department in the world was founded in 1930 by Leo Kanner (1894–1981), an Austrian immigrant and medical graduate of the University of Berlin, under the direction of Adolf Meyer at the Johns Hopkins Hospital, Baltimore, Maryland in the United States. Kanner was the first physician to be identified as a child psychiatrist in the United States; his textbook, *Child Psychiatry* (1935), is credited with introducing both the specialty and the term *Anglophone* to the academic community.[4] In 1936, Kanner established the first formal elective course in child psychiatry at the Johns Hopkins Hospital.[4]

American child psychiatry took root in 1909 when Jane Addams and her colleagues established the Juvenile Psychopathic Institute in Chicago, later renamed the Institute for Juvenile Research, and the world's first child guidance clinic.[5] William Healy, a neurologist by training, was its first director and was charged with not only studying the delinquent patients biological aspects of brain functioning and IQ but also their attitudes, motivations, and the impact of social factors.

From its establishment in February 1923, The Maudsley, a London-based postgraduate teaching and research psychiatric hospital, started a small psychiatry department for children.[6] Similar overall early developments took place in many other countries during the late 1920s and 1930. In the United States, CAP was established as a recognized medical specialty in 1953 with the founding of the American Academy of Child Psychiatry but was not established as a legitimate, board-certifiable medical specialty by the American Board of Psychiatry and Neurology until 1959.

Although the field has now been formally and firmly established in academic medicine for more than 50 years, the demand for child and adolescent psychiatrists continues to far outstrip the supply worldwide. There is also a severe maldistribution of child and adolescent psychiatrists, especially in rural and poor, urban areas where access is significantly reduced.[7,8] For example, there are currently only approximately 8700 practicing child and adolescent psychiatrists in the United States. A report by the US Bureau of Health Professions (2000) projected a need in the year 2020 for 12,624 child and adolescent psychiatrists.

The same report also stated that only 20% of emotionally disturbed children and adolescents received any mental health treatment, a tiny percentage of which was performed by child and adolescent psychiatrists. This concern is magnified manifold in lower- and middle-income (LAMI) countries, where there may only be a handful of child psychiatrists for a whole country. With no end in sight to the dearth of child and adolescent psychiatrists, not to mention child and adolescent behavioral health providers in other disciplines, organized child psychiatry and international organizations are not only focusing on traditional training of specialists but also on innovative training programs to build capacity of health personnel at different levels of medical training as well as in other fields.

This article outlines existing CAP training programs in different parts of the world and how they seek to address the growing need for trained CAP mental health personnel.

CHILD AND ADOLESCENT PSYCHIATRY IN THE UNITED STATES

As stated previously, the shortage of specialists in CAP necessary to meet current and projected clinical demands has been recognized for more than 15 years. Over the past decade, the American Academy of Child and Adolescent Psychiatry Task Force on Work Force Needs has examined some of the reasons for this shortage, which include inadequate support for CAP in academic institutions, limited graduate medical education funding, lower clinical revenues under a managed care environment, and a devalued image of the profession.[9] By the group's conservative estimates, even if funding and recruitment were to remain stable at the current levels, there would be 4312 fewer child and adolescent psychiatrists by the year 2020 than needed to maintain the (already suboptimal) 1995 use levels.[10] Recruitment and edification of multiple levels of trainees in pediatric mental health has, thus, been an organized priority in the health sector, especially in the past 2 decades.

UNDERGRADUATE MEDICAL EDUCATION

In most countries, the number of child and adolescent psychiatrists with academic appointments is limited; CAP programs are developed and taught by a small number of teaching staff in medical school. A survey done in the Australian medical schools found that approximately 4 to 12 hours were allotted for child psychiatry teaching at most schools, and clinical rotations were offered as an elective.[11] Even within the United States, there is limited agreement about curricula content for undergraduate CAP teaching programs in medical schools, with a wide range of objectives identified by different programs. On average, the time allowed for teaching CAP is limited. There is also great variation in the time allocated by different medical schools.[12]

Medical schools should reconsider the relatively low priority given to teaching CAP to medical students. The CAP profession must identify clear learning goals for a longitudinal developmentally appropriate model of CAP education commencing at an undergraduate level in medical schools and continuing through residency and fellowships. There is a need to promote national and international standards for teaching in this area and to encourage stronger collaborations between teaching staff across different medical schools. The Yale Child Study Center has been a leader in developing creative curricular initiatives before, during, and after medical school that address gaps in child mental health education, training, and recruitment challenges.[9] Several of these have been replicated through strategic collaborations with other institutions in the country.

GRADUATE TRAINING

In the United States, CAP training requires 4 years of medical school; at least 3 years of approved residency training in medicine, neurology, and general psychiatry with adults; and 2 years of additional specialized training in psychiatric work with children, adolescents, and their families in an accredited residency in CAP. Child and adolescent subspecialty training is similar in other Western countries (such as the United Kingdom, New Zealand, and Australia), in that trainees must generally demonstrate competency in general adult psychiatry before commencing subspecialty training in CAP.

There are several different training pathways to a career in CAP, each of which offers a unique training experience based on ones interests:

- *Traditional training programs*: Residents complete 5 total years of training: 3 years of general psychiatry residency training (including internship) plus 2 years of CAP specialty training.

The core competencies covered during the 5-year training period have been defined by the Accreditation Council of Graduate Medical Education (ACGME) through the psychiatry Residency Review Committee (RRC) (**Box 1**). Different programs have adopted varied teaching methodologies and learning schemas to deliver the knowledge and skills laid out by the psychiatry RRC.

For each period, review and reporting will involve selecting milestone levels that best describe each fellow's current performance and attributes. Milestones are arranged into numbered levels. Tracking from level 1 to level 5 is synonymous with moving from novice to expert in the subspecialty. These levels do not correspond with postgraduate year of education.

- *Integrated training programs*: Residents complete 5 years of training in general psychiatry and CAP at the same time.

An integrated training program provides training in adult and child psychiatry in a 5-year program. Unlike traditional training whereby adult psychiatry is completed before child training is begun, these programs allow for training in child psychiatry beginning in the first or second year of residency. For medical students who know that they want to become child psychiatrists, this is a good alternative path. Click here for a list of integrated programs.[13]

- *Triple board programs*: Triple board residents spend 5 years in an integrated training program focused on pediatrics, general psychiatry, and CAP. At the end of the training, residents are board eligible in all 3 disciplines.

Triple board graduates apply a developmentally informed, biopsychosocial approach to their work in health, illness, and prevention.

The training provides a foundation for excellence in clinical care, education, advocacy, public policy, and research.

Most importantly, triple board training transcends the traditional boundaries between pediatrics and psychiatry to allow graduates to optimize the medical care of children, adults, and families.

- *Post Pediatric Portal Program (PPPP)*: This training pathway is specifically designed for board-certified pediatricians who then choose to train as a child and adolescent

Box 1
The CAP core competencies

All CAP training programs must incorporate the general 6 core competencies mandated by ACGME. These core competencies include

- Patient care
- Medical knowledge
- Practice-based learning and improvement
- Interpersonal and communication skills
- Professionalism
- Systems-based practice

Note: In 2014, the ACGME published The Child & Adolescent Psychiatry Milestones. The milestones are designed only for use in the evaluation of resident physicians in the context of their participation in an ACGME-accredited residency or fellowship programs. The milestones provide a framework for the assessment of the development of the resident physician in key dimensions of the elements of physician competency in a specialty or subspecialty. They neither represent the entirety of the dimensions of the 6 domains of physician competency nor are they designed to be relevant in any other content.

The milestones are designed for programs to use in semiannual review of fellow performance and reporting to the ACGME. The milestones are knowledge, skills, attitudes, and other attributes for each of the ACGME competencies organized in a developmental framework from less to more advanced. They are descriptors and targets for fellow performance as a fellow moves from entry into fellowship through graduation. In the initial years of implementation, the review committee will examine milestone performance data for each program's fellows as one element in the Next Accreditation System to determine whether fellows overall are progressing.

Data from ACGME, ABPN. The Child & Adolescent Psychiatry Milestone Project. 2014. Available at: http://www.acgme.org/acgmeweb/Portals/0/PDFs/Milestones/ChildandAdolescentPsychiatryMilestones.pdf. Accessed November 30, 2014.

psychiatrist. The program is a 3-year training experience in general psychiatry and in CAP that creates an abbreviated pathway between pediatrics and psychiatry. The PPPP project began in 2007 as an effort to provide an efficient way for pediatricians to train in CAP. To date, 5 programs offer this training in the United States.

CERTIFICATION AND CONTINUING EDUCATION

In the United States, having completed the CAP residency, the child and adolescent psychiatrist is eligible to take the additional certification examination in the subspecialty of CAP from the American Board of Psychiatry and Neurology (ABPN) or the American Osteopathic Board of Neurology and Psychiatry (AOBNP) if the resident graduates from an osteopathic medical school.[14] Although the ABPN and AOBNP examinations are not required for practice, they are a further assurance that the child and adolescent psychiatrist with these certifications can be expected to diagnose and treat all psychiatric conditions in patients of any age competently. Training requirements are listed on the Web site of The American Academy of Child and Adolescent Psychiatry.[15]

CHILD AND ADOLESCENT PSYCHIATRY IN EUROPE

The development and training in the subspecialty of CAP in Europe hails from diverse historical traditions as outlined in Remschmidt and van Engeland's[16] excellent historical overview of the discipline across diverse European countries. The historical streams include the neuropsychiatric, remedial clinical, psychoanalytic and empirical, epidemiologic, and statistical traditions depending on specific countries.[16] For instance, teaching psychiatry alongside neurology was an established practice in several countries, including many Eastern European countries, Germany, Italy, and some establishments in France. The remedial or defectology tradition flourished in Austria and Switzerland, practices established by the founding fathers Hans Asperger and Paul Moore, respectively, and was also popular in some Eastern European countries. The psychoanalytic training influences were prevalent and still persist in Western Europe, whereas the research- and evidence-based influences stemming from the birth of academic CAP took hold in the United Kingdom, the Scandinavian countries, the Netherlands, and some German institutions.[17]

More than 90% of European countries have national organizations representing CAP. In more than half of the European countries, CAP training organizations are part of general psychiatric organizations. However, there are still some European countries where there are no formal training programs in CAP.[17] Attempts to unify clinical practice and training across Europe date back to the establishment of the European scientific and professional international organizations as far back as the first symposium of the European Child and Adolescent Psychiatrists in Switzerland in 1954 and currently the European Society for Child and Adolescent Psychiatry.

UNDERGRADUATE TRAINING

The level of undergraduate training in medical school varies from short occasional seminars to more structured training programs involving clinical placements and practicum. However, many medical schools and faculties still do not have independent academic departments or formal undergraduate teaching programs in their medical schools. Where academic CAP departments do exist, teaching of CAP usually takes place either as part of general psychiatry or as part of the pediatric modules and blocks of time teaching.

POSTGRADUATE TRAINING

One of the early surveys of CAP training in Europe established that CAP is not a specialty in its own right in about a third of European countries and that the length of training varied between 12 and 96 months with different entry requirements into the CAP training scheme across countries.[18]

It is often thought that postgraduate training is aligned with adult psychiatry. However, in a recent survey conducted in 34 counties, only 7 out of 28 responding countries reported a common pathway via general psychiatry to training in CAP.[17] Finland and Germany have the best-developed independent CAP curriculum whereby trainees can choose to specialize in CAP early on in their careers.[17]

Despite some commonalities, there is huge variation across Europe in resources devoted to the specialty, including the number of existing child and adolescent psychiatrists, the number of trainees entering the profession, the structure of training, the organization of services and clinical and research practice, with all components of the CAP profession continuing to be influenced by respective historical traditions and context. In some countries, despite relatively adequate numbers of adult psychiatrists, there is a lack of interest in additional training in CAP,[19] possibly because of few job opportunities. This case is particularly true in Eastern Europe. With the sound establishment of academic CAP over the last several decades, the empirical, biological, and epidemiologic approach to the profession is superseding hitherto established traditions with an evidence-based approach to training and practice.

THE EUROPEAN UNION OF MEDICAL SPECIALISTS: THE EUROPEAN UNION OF MEDICAL SPECIALISTS CURRICULUM FOR CHILD AND ADOLESCENT PSYCHIATRY

The ever-closer links between countries and institutions have resulted in a quest for increased standardization and quality improvement in the training of all medical specialties across Europe; more recently, the same applies to CAP. The European Union of Medical Specialists (UEMS) is a nongovernmental organization representing national associations of medical specialists at the European level. Its aims include the improvement of medical training and, consequently, the promotion of free movement of European physicians. Since 2005, following the directive of the European Parliament, the European Union countries now mutually recognize each other's medical qualifications.[20]

At the same time, the UEMS is dedicated to establishing the highest standards of training and care for the benefit of the patients. The UEMS covers the areas of continuing medical education, postgraduate training, and quality assurance.[20] The UEMS guidelines for training are not meant to override individual countries curricula, but there is an expectation that the joint curriculum will enhance the quality of training overall.

THE MAIN PRINCIPLES UNDERLYING THE EUROPEAN UNION OF MEDICAL SPECIALISTS CHILD AND ADOLESCENT PSYCHIATRY TRAINING

The curriculum consists of sections on the content of training, the theoretic knowledge and the practical skills and professionalism required by trainees, the actual organization of training, and the minimum credentials required for the trainers. The UEMS recommends that all curricula should have national approval and be regularly audited by the relevant government authority responsible for education and training.

The length of training is recommended to take a minimum of 3 years. The *UEMS Log Book*[21] makes the following specific recommendations of mandatory requirements: "Goals to be acquired to a high level of skill by all trainees by the time they are recognized as a qualified child and adolescent psychiatrist."[21] These goals are as follows:

- Establishing and maintaining therapeutic relationships with children and adolescents of all ages and with families
- Knowledge of normal child development and milestones
- Safeguarding and knowledge of the legal framework
- Assessment and diagnosis of children and adolescents who have mental health problems using a biopsychosocial model
- Knowledge of culture and diversity influences
- Mental health emergencies
- Use of medication and limitations of psychoactive medicines for children and adolescents
- Psychological interventions
- Neurologic examination and tests
- Neuropsychiatry including attention-deficit/hyperactivity disorder, autism, seizures, and the impact of other developmental and brain disorders on the mental health of children and adolescents; inpatient child or adolescent services
- Research

- Knowledge of service pathways
- Knowledge of networks involving other colleagues in medicine and with multi-agency networks

According to the *UEMS Log Book*, the goals that are required AT a basic minimum level but that may not be obtained AT a specialist level by the time the trainee is recognized as a qualified child and adolescent psychiatrist, are as follows[20]:

- Mental health of infants and children younger than 5 years
- Specialize in adolescent psychiatry and the transition to adult mental health services
- Adolescent forensic psychiatry
- Anxiety disorders
- Disruptive behavior disorders
- Obsessional compulsive disorder
- Depression
- Psychosis
- Bipolar disorders
- Eating disorders
- Emerging personality disorders
- Work with traumatized children and adolescents and their families (eg, war, natural disasters, and so forth)
- Substance misuse
- Pediatric liaison psychiatry
- Psychosomatic disorders and conversion phenomena
- Learning disability/mental impairment (handicap)
- Quality assurance–service development
- Management and leadership
- Teaching
- Medicolegal work
- Ethics as applied to child mental health

POSTGRADUATE TRAINING IN CHILD AND ADOLESCENT PSYCHIATRY IN THE UNITED KINGDOM

The Royal College of Psychiatrists is the professional and educational body for psychiatrists in the United Kingdom.[22,23] The Postgraduate Education Services Section of the college in conjunction with the network of the pertinent medical school/university deans oversee the registration and training of all core and specialty trainees in accordance with the General Medical Council (GMC) standards.

Training is program based and time limited. Advanced training opportunities are offered and are individually tailored; movement into and out of training and between training programs is facilitated, depending on individual trainee's requirements, career plans, and development.

The curriculum, assessment, and appraisal processes are aimed at the successful fulfillment of core competencies achieved in the work place, accreditation through the examination system, and enhancement of continued professional development and reflective practice. More specifically, in order to practice as a psychiatrist, a doctor must complete a full 6-year program of GMC-approved training in psychiatry and pass all sections of the Membership of the Royal College of Psychiatrists (MRCPsych) Examination. The training includes 3 years at core training level followed by 3 years at an advanced and/or higher training level in a GMC-approved training program. The award of a Certificate of Completed Training is given to doctors who complete an approved program of psychiatry and pass all sections of the MRCPsych Examinations. A normal training program would consist of

- A minimum of 36 months whole time equivalent in core training also referred to as general psychiatric training (CT1–CT3)
- Completion of at least 36 months whole time equivalent in advanced training (ST4–ST6)

THE UNITED KINGDOM–CHILD AND ADOLESCENT PSYCHIATRY CURRICULUM

The new advanced training curriculum in CAP was launched in 2013, after soliciting wide input from a variety of stakeholders, including young people.[23] The curriculum includes core and specialty competencies and research requirements. The core competencies cover mandatory intended learning objectives (ILOs) and selective ILOs.

The United Kingdom mandatory intended learning objectives are as follows:

- Professionalism
- Establishing therapeutic relationships with children, adolescents, and families
- Safeguarding children
- Undertaking clinical assessment
- Managing emergencies
- Pediatric psychopharmacology
- Psychological therapies
- Assessment and treatment of child and adolescent neuropsychiatry
- Working with networks
- Teaching and supervision and lifelong networks
- Management for all

Given the current breadth and wealth of knowledge of CAP, not all trainees will have the opportunity to train in every aspect of the profession or indeed work in every setting. Ideally, all trainees should work in a child and adolescent inpatient setting and day-treatment setting. It is usually common to establish regional training opportunities for those aspects of the curriculum that are difficult to organize locally, for instance, training in substance abuse, learning disabilities, pediatric liaison consultation work, specific research activities, and some psychological therapies.

All trainees have access to regular assessments of their progress in training and supervision. The mechanisms for assessment have become much more practice based and take place in the clinical setting. The Annual Review of Competence Progression is a formal process applied to all specialty trainees, including CAP trainees. The process establishes whether a trainee can progress to the next stage of their training.

THE EXPERIENCES OF TRAINEES IN EUROPE

Simmons and colleagues[17] (2012) conducted a survey of trainee experiences of CAP training across Europe with respect to training quality and content, working conditions, and recruitment. Twenty-eight out of 34 countries with CAP training programs responded to the survey. The data were validated by the UEMS CAP group and trainees of the 2011 CAP forum of the European Federation of Psychiatric trainees (EFPT), a nonprofit making overarching organization established in Utrecht in 1993. The EFPT's central activity is aimed at improving the quality of education across Europe.

In the same survey it was established that standardized assessments of trainees' progress and access to supervision arrangements vary across Europe, but it would seem that in most countries supervision is obligatory. Psychotherapy training, including psychodynamic training and cognitive-behavioral therapy, takes place in two-thirds of countries across Europe; but there is still a dearth of practical psychotherapy training. In some countries, self-analysis remains obligatory. In view of the profession becoming more evidence based, it is of concern that only a third of training programs regard research as an obligatory training experience. Working conditions for trainees are broadly similar across European countries with salaries that are comparable with those in adult psychiatry and pediatrics; but in some countries, access to part-time work is not available. It would seem that recruitment to such positions is a universal problem following the completion of CAP training.[17]

CHILD AND ADOLESCENT PSYCHIATRY IN OTHER PARTS OF THE WORLD

In comparison with Europe and North America, relatively little is reported regarding CAP training in the other parts of the world. Certain regions of Asia and Africa constitute some of the most dynamic and rapidly developing world regions with very young populations. A study conducted by Morris and colleagues[24] reflected an overall scarcity of child mental health services and a mental health gap in which LAMI countries lag significantly behind high-income countries. This study also reported a higher rate of unmet needs in child mental health training in LAMI countries. In an article focused on West and South Asian countries, Srinath and colleagues[25] reported that, in comparison with Europe and North America, there have been huge unmet needs for CAP resources in Asia, notwithstanding the rapidly growing numbers of youngsters who require mental health evaluation and ongoing care. Some child and adolescent mental health graduate training programs have been established in individual universities in South East Asia and Africa, like the one at the National Institute of Mental Health and Neurosciences in Bangalore, India and also at the University of Ibadan in Nigeria. However, the presence and availability of such institutions are rare.

CHILD AND ADOLESCENT PSYCHIATRY TRAINING IN THE FAR EAST

At this point, there is relatively little published about CAP needs and about CAP training and academic CAP in regions of the Far East. The Far East, however, is one of the most dynamic and rapidly developing regions in the world, with a very young population. Within the past 2 decades, several articles have reported emerging needs related to the paucity of child and adolescent mental health (CAMH) resources in several Far East countries.[3–8,26] More recently published articles on CAP training in Hong Kong, Malaysia, Singapore, and Japan reported severe workforce shortages in CAMH services.[27–32]

In order to investigate CAP needs and map and optimize training programs for future workforce development in this region, the Consortium on Academic Child and Adolescent Psychiatry in the Far East (CACAP-FE) was established in 2011.[33] This consortium is supported by the World Psychiatry Association, Section on Child and Adolescent Psychiatry, Group on Teaching and Learning. Through this consortium, information was gathered regarding the potential future implications for CAP training in the Far East region.

For the purposes of this article, the Far East region is described as including the following 20 countries that are functionally self-governing or specially administered areas: Brunei, Cambodia, People's Republic of China (China), East Timor, Hong Kong (technically a Special Administrative Region of the People's Republic of China),

Indonesia, Japan, Lao People's Democratic Republic (Lao PDR), Macau (technically a Special Administrative Region of the People's Republic of China), Malaysia, Myanmar, Mongolia, North Korea, Philippines, Russian Far East Region (Russia), Singapore, South Korea, Chinese Taipei (also known as Taiwan, though not a recognized distinct country by the United Nations), Thailand, and Vietnam.

Leading academic child and adolescent psychiatrists in the Far East were invited to join the consortium (CACAP-FE). There were no objections or refusals expressed in participating in the CACAP-FE; it included faculty within leading universities, some of whom were also representatives of specialty societies within the identified Far East countries and areas. The consortium members provided information on current CAP postgraduate training and education systems via an internally distributed questionnaire administered over a period of 10 weeks. Information was then organized and its accuracy checked by the authors. The initial questionnaire was created by the CACAP-FE board and piloted with input from 5 countries in the Far East. The questionnaire was composed in English and included the following questions:

1. How many qualified (board-certified) general psychiatrists are there?
2. How many of the general psychiatrists treat child and adolescent populations?
3. Is there a national guideline for postgraduate general psychiatry training?
4. What is the duration of general psychiatry training?
5. Is there any CAP exposure during general psychiatry training and, if so, how long?
6. Is CAP recognized as a separate specialty (subspecialty)?
7. Is there a specialized postgraduate training program in CAP and, if so, how long?
8. Is there a national guideline for postgraduate CAP training?
9. Are overseas CAP electives available for trainees and, if so, in which countries?
10. Is there a need for more child and adolescent psychiatrists (and/or child adolescent mental health specialists)?
11. If so, what are the estimated numbers of required CAMH professionals?
12. How many CAP departments affiliated to universities are there?
13. Is there a CAP society?
14. Is there a national CAP journal?
15. Is there a national child and adolescent mental health policy?

The survey did not include questions as to the content of CAP training, with an assumption that limited numbers of included countries and areas had structured training systems. Information was provided by the consortium members, who represented 17 out of 20 identified countries and areas in the Far East (East Timor, North Korea, and Macau were not represented). Information is summarized in **Table 1**. At the time of the study, the number of qualified psychiatrists ranged from 2 in Lao PDR to 21,500 in China. Similarly, the number of psychiatrists treating youth also varied from one in Brunei to most of the qualified psychiatrists (numbering 13,534) in Japan. National guidelines for general psychiatry residency training existed in 11 out of 17 countries and areas. The duration of this training varied from 12 months in Mongolia and Russia to 72 months in Hong Kong (median: 36 months). In 16 countries and areas, a mandatory examination was required to graduate from the training program. CAP rotations were available for trainees during general psychiatry residency in 12 out of 17 countries and areas (median: 3 months; range: 2 to 6 months). Some trainees were able to experience CAP electives in other foreign countries, such as Australia, Canada, the United Kingdom, and the United States.

CAP was not recognized as a subspecialty in 5 countries (Japan, Lao PDR, Myanmar, Russia, and Singapore). CAP postgraduate training was available in

Table 1
Countries and areas with their characteristics

Country	N of Qualified Psychiatrists	N of Psychiatrists Treating Youth	National Guideline for Psychiatry Training	Duration of Training (mo)	CAP Recognized as Subspecialty (y)	CAP Exposure During General Training	CAP Postgraduate Training	National Guideline for CAP Training	Duration of CAP Training (mo)
Brunei	4	1	NR	NR	Y (2005)	NR	N	N	—
Cambodia	41	NR	Y	36	Y (1996)	NR	N	N	—
China	20,500	500	Y	36	Y (1980)	Y (2 mo)	Y	N	36
Hong Kong	300	30	N	>72	Y	Y (6 mo)	N	N	—
Indonesia	600	40	N	24	Y (1978)	Y (6 mo)	Y	N	12
Japan	13,534	Most psychiatrists	Y	60	N	N	Y	N	>36
Lao PDR	2	2	N	NR	N	NR	N	N	—
Malaysia	289	>25	Y	18 or 36	Y	Y (4 mo)	Y	Y	18 or 36
Myanmar	80	80	Y	24	N	Y (2 mo)	N	N	—
Mongolia	135	2	Y	12	Y (1978)	Y (2 mo)	N	N	—
Philippines	400	20	Y	36–48	Y (1972)	Y (3 mo)	Y	Y	24
Russia	509	72	Y	12–24	N	Y (4 mo)	Y	N	1–4
Singapore	150	25	Y	36	N	Y (6 mo)	Y	N	12
South Korea	200	>400	N	48	Y (1980)	Y (2 mo)	Y	N	24
Taiwan	1400	400	Y	48	Y (1998)	Y (3 mo)	Y	Y	12
Thailand	520	120	Y	36	Y	Y (3 mo)	Y	Y	48
Vietnam	700	10	N	>24	Y	N	N	N	—

Country	CAP Electives in Overseas	Need for More CAP Specialists	Estimated N of Specialists Required	N of Academic CAP Departments	CAP Society	CAP Scientific National Journal	National CAMH Policy	Income Level[a]
Brunei	N	Y	>2	0	N	N	N	High
Cambodia	N	Y	5–10	0	Y	N	N	Low
China	AU, UK, USA	Y	8000	15	Y	N	Y	Upper-middle
Hong Kong	N	Y	20–30	2	N	N	N	High
Indonesia	N	Y	7000	0	Y	N	Y	Lower-middle
Japan	UK, USA	Y	NN	1	Y	Y	Y	High
Lao PDR	N	Y	51	0	N	N	N	Lower-middle
Malaysia	AU, UK	Y	NN	0	Y	N	Y	Upper-middle
Myanmar	N	Y	NN	0	N	N	N	Low
Mongolia	South Korea	NR	NN	0	N	N	Y	Lower-middle
Philippines	N	Y	50	1	Y	N	Y	Lower-middle
Russia	N	Y	26	0	Y	N	N	High
Singapore	AU, UK, USA	Y	NN	2	N	N	N	High
South Korea	UK, USA	Y	200	30	Y	Y	N	High
Chinese Taipei	UK, USA	Y	200	10	Y	N	Y	High[b]
Thailand	UK, Singapore	Y	100	0	Y	N	Y	Upper-middle
Vietnam	N	Y	100	0	N	N	N	Lower-middle

Abbreviations: AU, Australia; N, no; NN, not known; Y, yes.

[a] Based on the data from World Bank.

[b] The data of Taiwan are not separated from that of China, but it is considered to be a high-income country per World Bank Web site.

Data from Hirota T, Guerrero A, Sartorius N, et al. Consortium on Academic Child and Adolescent Psychiatry in the Far East (CACAP FE). Child and adolescent psychiatry in the Far East. Psychiatry Clin Neurosci 2015;69(3):171–7; and Remschmidt H, van Engeland H, editors. Child and adolescent psychiatry in Europe, historical development, current situation and future perspectives. Darmstadt (Germany); New York: Steinkopff; Springer; 1999.

10 countries and areas, whereas national guidelines for CAP training existed only in 4 countries and areas. Among 10 countries and areas that provided data, the duration of CAP training varied from 12 to 48 months (median: 30 months). When countries were classified by income level based on data from the World Bank,[16] of note, CAP was recognized as a subspecialty only in 50% (3 out of 6) of high-income countries and areas, whereas it was recognized as a subspecialty in all (9 out of 9) middle-income countries. Furthermore, national guidelines for CAP postgraduate training existed only in Chinese Taipei (Taiwan) out of 4 high-income places in comparison with 3 middle-income countries (Malaysia, Philippines, and Thailand).

Shortage of CAP specialists was apparent, despite local needs, from the data of all countries and areas except for Mongolia (data not reported). Sixteen countries and areas estimated minimal numbers of required CAP specialists, which varied from 2 in Brunei to 8000 in China. In 8 of the 17 included countries and areas, a national child and adolescent mental health policy was available. With regard to academic CAP, the results were not particularly encouraging, as there were, among the 17 countries and areas, relatively small numbers with university-affiliated academic CAP departments (7 countries and areas; range was one in Japan and the Philippines to 30 in South Korea); a national CAP society (10 countries and areas); and national CAP scientific journals (2 countries and areas).

This survey is the first survey to recognize and map current child and adolescent mental health services and CAP training system in the Far East region. It revealed overall underdevelopment of postgraduate CAP training system and a resultant scarcity of services despite the awareness of unmet needs and CAP's recognition as a subspecialty in 12 of 17 countries and areas.

SUMMARY

The development of the specialty of CAP extends back to the late nineteenth and beginning of the twentieth century in line with many advances in general psychiatry. Different traditions and cultural contexts occasioned the development and maintenance of theoretic models and practice of CAP depending on the teaching at the time and the influences exerted by the leaders in the profession. With ever-closer links at all levels across Europe and the United States, the last couple of decades have seen a quest for the standardization of teaching and training, all in the interests of children and young people and their families and the profession.

The standardization of practice is exemplified in the UEMS curriculum whose basic principles are set out. The outlined curriculum aims at producing CAP professionals who perform at the highest level with excellent outcomes, who are good communicators and collaborators, managers of their services, and an ardent health advocate with a sustained interest in research and the advancement of their profession. These competencies set forth by the UEMS curriculum are not very different in their content than that outlined by the ACGME and the psychiatry RRC in the United States. CAP psychiatrists, at the end of their training, will aim to continue their professional development. They will be capable of working in a team and will exercise a professional attitude toward patients and families. CAP psychiatrists will possess integrity and probity and promote health values through research and teaching. CAP training programs in the LAMI countries are sprouting with impressive creativity (given minimal resources), cultural applicability, acceptability, and outcomes. Some of these are mainly focused on capacity-building curricula in child mental health that target general physicians, pediatricians, school teachers, as well as community and lady health workers that work in communities at the ground level. Child psychiatry training programs not only offer training in teaching the clinical skills of the discipline of CAP but also strive to help with the development of professionalism, ethical behaviors, and leadership skills in their trainees. Ultimately, it is the children of the world who stand to gain by having a skilled work force that adheres to the highest global standards when it comes to the provision of mental health services.

REFERENCES

1. Gerhard UJ, Schönberg A, Blanz B. Johannes Trüper–mediator between child and adolescent psychiatry and pedagogy. Z Kinder Jugendpsychiatr Psychother 2008;36(1):55–63.
2. Nissen G. Hermann Emminghaus. Founder of scientific child adolescent and psychiatry. Z Kinder Jugendpsychiatr 1986;14(1):81–7 [in German].
3. Eliasberg WG. In memoriam: Moritz Tramer M.D. (1882-1963). Am J Psychiatry 1964;121:103–4.
4. Available at: http://www.hopkinsmedicine.org/psychiatry/specialty_areas/child_adolescent/. Accessed November 30, 2014.
5. Beuttler F, Bell C. For the welfare of every child – a brief history of the Institute for Juvenile Research, 1909–2010. Chicago: University of Illinois; 2010.
6. Evans B, Rahman S, Jones E. Managing the 'unmanageable': interwar child psychiatry at the Maudsley Hospital, London. Hist Psychiatry 2008;19(4): 454–75.
7. Thomas CR, Holzer CE. The continuing shortage of child and adolescent psychiatrists,. J Am Acad Child Adolesc Psychiatry 2006;45(9):1023–31.
8. Belfer ML. Child and adolescent mental disorders: the magnitude of the problem across the globe. J Child Psychol Psychiatry 2008;49:226–36.
9. Martin A, Bloch M, Pruett K, et al. From too little too late to early and often: child psychiatry education during medical school (and before and after). Child Adolesc Psychiatr Clin N Am 2007;16:17–43.
10. Kim WJ. Child and adolescent psychiatry workforce: a critical shortage and national challenge. Acad Psychiatry 2003;27(4):277–82.
11. Sawyer M, Giesen F. Undergraduate teaching of child and adolescent psychiatry in Australia: survey of current practice. Aust N Z J Psychiatry 2007;41(8): 675–81.
12. Sawyer MG, Giesen F, Walter G. Child psychiatry curricula in undergraduate medical education. J Am Acad Child Adolesc Psychiatry 2008;47(2):139–47.
13. Available at: http://www.aacap.org/aacap/Medical_Students_and_Residents/Medical_Students/Integrated_Training_Programs.aspx. Accessed November 30, 2014.
14. Available at: http://en.wikipedia.org/wiki/American_Board_of_Psychiatry_and_Neurology. Accessed November 30, 2014.
15. Available at: http://www.aacap.org/aacap/Medical_Students_and_Residents/Residents_and_Fellows/Child_and_Adolescent_Psychiatry_Training.aspx. Accessed November 30, 2014.
16. Remschmidt H, van Engeland H, editors. Child and adolescent psychiatry in Europe, historical development, current situation and future perspectives. Darmstadt (Germany); New York: Springer; Steinkopff; 1999.
17. Simmons M, Barrett E, Wilkinson P, et al. Trainee experiences of child and adolescent psychiatry (CAP) training in Europe: 2010-2011 survey of the European Federation of Psychiatric Trainees (EFPT) CAP working group. Eur Child Adolesc Psychiatry 2012;21:433–42.

18. Karabekiroglu K, Dogangun B, Herguner S, et al. Child and adolescent psychiatry training in Europe: differences and challenges in harmonization. Eur Child Adolesc Psychiatry 2006;15(18):467–75.
19. World Health Organization. Child and adolescent atlas: resources for child and adolescent mental health. Geneva (United Kingdom): World Health Organization; 2005.
20. European Union of Medical Specialists (UEMS). Training requirements for the specialty of child and adolescent psychiatry, European standards of postgraduate medical specialist training. 2014. Available at: www.uems.net. Accessed December 17, 2014.
21. European training log-book for child and adolescent psychiatry (UEMS). 2014. Available at: UEMS_Logbook_final__-_12-01-2014_-_no_password-2.pdf. Accessed July 24, 2015.
22. Specialist training in psychiatry. A comprehensive guide to training and assessment in the UK for trainees and local educational providers, occasional paper OP 69. London: The Royal College of Psychiatrists; 2010.
23. A competency based curriculum for specialist training in psychiatry. Specialists in child an adolescent psychiatry. London: Royal College of Psychiatrists; 2010 (Updated March 2012), © Royal College of Psychiatrists.
24. Morris J, Belfer M, Daniels A, et al. Treated prevalence of and mental health services received by children and adolescents in 42 low-and-middle-income countries. J Child Psychol Psychiatry 2011;52(12):1239–46.
25. Srinath S, Kandasamy P, Golhar TS. Epidemiology of child and adolescent mental health disorders in Asia. Curr Opin Psychiatry 2010;23(4):330–6.
26. Manheimer M. Les troubles mentaux de l'enfance (review). J Ment Sci 1900; 46(193):342–3.
27. McClure M, Shirataki S. Child psychiatry in Japan. J Am Acad Child Adolesc Psychiatry 1989;28(4):488–92.
28. McClure GM. Child and family psychiatry in China. J Am Acad Child Adolesc Psychiatry 1987;26(5):806–10.
29. Mckelvey RS, Sang DL, Tu HC. Is there a role for child psychiatry in Vietnam? Aust N Z J Psychiatry 1997;31(1):114–9.
30. WongCK. Child psychiatry in Hong Kong: an overview. Aust N Z J Psychiatry 1990;24(3):331–8.
31. Tan S, Fung D, Hung SF, et al. Growing wealth and growing pains: child and adolescent psychiatry in Hong Kong, Malaysia and Singapore. Australas Psychiatry 2008;16(3):204–9.
32. Tateno M, Uchida N, Kikuchi S, et al. The practice of child and adolescent psychiatry: a survey of early-career psychiatrists in Japan. Child Adolesc Psychiatry Ment Health 2009;3(1):30.
33. Hirota T, Guerrero A, Sartorius N, et al, Consortium on Academic Child and Adolescent Psychiatry in the Far East (CACAP FE). Child and adolescent psychiatry in the Far East. Psychiatry Clin Neurosci 2015;69(3):171–7.

Displaced Children

The Psychological Implications

Paramjit T. Joshi, MD[a,*], John A. Fayyad, MD[b]

KEYWORDS

• War • Displacement • Refugees • Exile • Children

KEY POINTS

- Millions of people across the world have been displaced or live in exile and/or as refugees largely as a consequence of wars, acts of terrorism, and catastrophic natural disasters.
- Today, more than ever before, cities, villages, and towns in many parts of the world have become battlefields, and children are the ones who get caught in the cross fire.
- The effects of overwhelming and inescapable stressors are challenging and complex for children whose age and psychological immaturity render them extremely vulnerable.
- The often intertwined contributions of psychosocial, economic, political, cultural, religious, and community variables have come to be appreciated as confounding factors having an enormous psychological impact.
- Children may be provided food, shelter, and clothing and have their medical needs attended to, but their emotional and psychological needs go unrecognized and unmet, with dire and monumental long-term consequences.

INTRODUCTION

Today, more than ever before, cities, villages, and towns in many parts of the world have become battlefields, and children are the ones who get caught in the cross fire. Regardless of the specific character of any particular war or act of terror or a natural disaster that often involve large numbers of victims to be displaced, such circumstances by definition involve destruction, pain, and death. Although these physical losses can be reconstructed or replaced, with the accompanying pain and sorrow gradually diminishing, the psychological scars, the trauma and the horrifying images and memories, do not heal as easily. These experiences are perhaps most challenging and complex for children whose age and psychological immaturity render them more

---

Conflicts: None.

[a] Department of Psychiatry & Behavioral Sciences, Children's National Medical Center, George Washington University School of Medicine, 111 Michigan Avenue Northwest, Floor 2.5 West, Suite 700, Washington, DC 20010, USA; [b] Faculty of Medicine, St George Hospital, University Medical Center, Balamand University, Institute for Development, Research, Advocacy and Applied Care (IDRAAC), Beirut, Lebanon

* Corresponding author.

E-mail address: PJOSHI@childrensnational.org

Child Adolesc Psychiatric Clin N Am 24 (2015) 715–730

http://dx.doi.org/10.1016/j.chc.2015.06.003 childpsych.theclinics.com vulnerable to the effects of overwhelming and inescapable stressors. It has generally been found that the psychological effects related to war and terrorism are quite similar to those associated with natural and man-initiated disastrous events, and the often intertwined contributions of psychosocial, economic, political, cultural, religious, and community variables have come to be appreciated as confounding factors having an enormous psychological impact.

There are now more than 50 million displaced people, the highest figure since World War II (United Nations [UN] Report 2013).[1] The wars in Syria and South Sudan and the conflicts in the Central African Republic, Iraq, Kenya, and Afghanistan have all added to these alarming numbers. There are now a staggering number of refugees, asylum seekers, and displaced people (**Fig. 1**). It has not been that high since the post-World War II era, when half the globe or more was dislocated.[1]

Half of the displaced are children, according to a UN refugee agency report.[1] The annual report, released by the UN High Commission for Refugees (UNHCR), showed a jump of 6 million people from 2012 to 2013. The massive increase was attributed to the war in Syria and the displacement in the Central African Republic and South Sudan. The war in Syria has resulted in 2.5 million refugees and has displaced 6.5 million people within the country, according to the report.

Afghans, Syrians, and Somalis accounted for more than half of the total refugees (**Fig. 2**). Pakistan, Iran, and Lebanon hosted more refugees than other countries. Most of the global forced displacement was internal displacement within countries, a record 33.3 million people and the largest increase in any group in the report.

In addition, more than 1 million submitted applications for asylum in 2013. A record number were children separated from parents. The year 2013 also saw one of the lowest levels of refugees returning home in 25 years. The UNHCR releases annual statistics showing that more than 51 million people were forcibly displaced at the end of 2013, the largest number since the end of World War II. Half of the world's refugees in 2013 were children.[1] An estimated 10.7 million individuals were newly displaced because of conflict or persecution in 2013. An average of 32,200 individuals per day were forced to leave their homes and seek protection elsewhere because of conflict and persecution in 2013. Lebanon hosted the most refugees in relation to its population, 178 registered refugees per 1000 inhabitants. These figures are likely to be

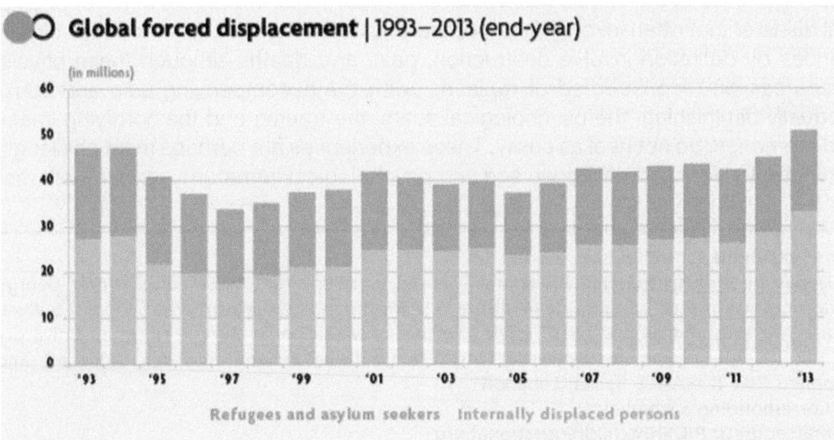

Fig. 1. Global forced displacement. (*From* United Nations High Commission for Refugees. Displacement: the new 21st century challenge. Geneva, Switzerland: UNHCR, 2013. Available at: http://www.unhcr.org.)

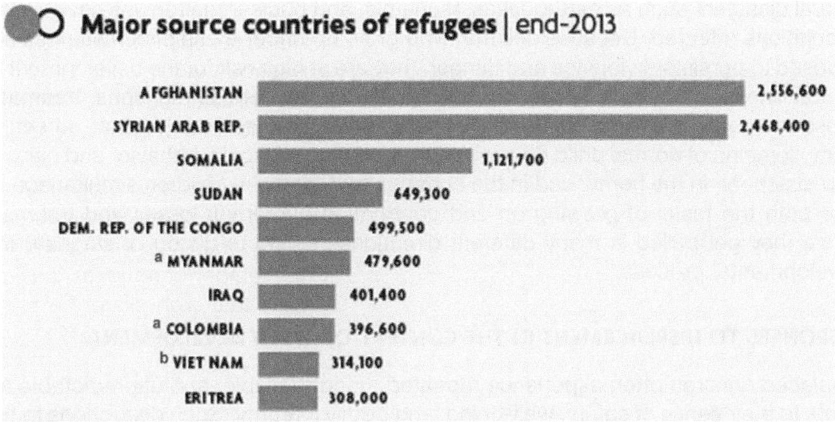

Fig. 2. Major source countries of refugees. [a]Includes people in a refugeelike situation. [b]The 300,000 Vietnamese refugees are well integrated and in practice receive protection from the Government of China. (*From* United Nations High Commission for Refugees. Displacement: the new 21st century challenge. Geneva, Switzerland: UNHCR, 2013. Available at: http://www.unhcr.org.)

underestimates because of large numbers of refugees who do not register with UNHCR for fear of retaliation by forces affiliated with the regimes from which they flee. More than 46% (5.4 million) of the refugees under UNHCR's mandate resided in countries where the gross domestic product per capita was less than $5000.

Often, little attention has been paid to the psychological well-being of displaced children who become victim to or a witness to such events. The resulting psychological impact results from the inability to predict, foresee, or even influence such events leading to a sense of hopelessness, helplessness, increased incidences of alcohol and drug use, violence, delinquency, and conduct problems. In an environment characterized by such suffering, deprivation, and conflict, the developmental aspects of childhood are severely affected. Displaced children are often exposed to trauma-related events that they are often forced to endure, leading to marked disruptions in the contextual and social fabric within which they live. Yet, few studies have examined the effects of war and terrorism on children. From the studies done during and after World War II[2] and the Yom Kippur War[3,4] to those documenting psychological outcomes from more recent wars,[5,6] it is evident that war experiences can hinder the psychosocial development of children and their expectations regarding future life. Evidence is emerging that war exposure during childhood has long-term adverse mental health outcomes. In Lebanon, a national survey revealed that 59% of children younger than 10 years and 84% of children and adolescents between 11 and 18 years were exposed to at least 1 war event. Experiencing war events before the age of 10 years increased the risk of developing a first-onset of anxiety and mood and impulse control disorders in later life.[7]

A circumscribed body of research during the last 2 decades has highlighted the various aspects of working with displaced populations and trauma work. The wars in the Balkans, Afghanistan, and the Middle East are good examples of the array of traumatic experiences victims who are displaced from their homes and communities and forced to live in refugee camps within their own countries (internally displaced) or endure exile, becoming refugees in other countries. The situations in other parts of the world such as South Africa, Southeast Asia, and Japan illustrate the strife war and natural disasters such as earthquakes, tsunamis, and nuclear meltdowns have on the populations affected. Because children who grow up under these circumstances are exposed to persistent violence and danger, they are at high risk for the development of mental illness. In addition to the expected posttraumatic stress reactions, traumatic stress can have an even more insidious impact in children and adolescents, affecting many domains of normal child development, including prosocial behavior and citizenship at school, in the home, and in the community. Displaced children simultaneously face both the tasks of growing up and confronting numerous losses and traumas. Often, they get pulled in many different directions serving to distort or stagnate the developmental process.[8]

RESPONSES TO DISPLACEMENT IN THE CONTEXT OF CHILD DEVELOPMENT

Displaced children often experience repeated, uncontrollable, and unpredictable affronts to their sense of safety, well-being, and bodily integrity. Such disruptions to the normal developmental trajectories of childhood can set into motion a cascade of effects on development. As children's brains, minds, and bodies change and grow over the course of their young lives, their reactions typically vary by age and developmental level. Therefore, it is important to view these reactions within the context of their social-cognitive processes occurring during each developmental stage.[8]

Preschool Years (<6 Years)

Children in the preschool years often have the most vague and somatic responses that may mask the magnitude of their distress.[9,10] Cognitively, children younger than 6 years have a difficult time taking others' perspectives. As a result, they often focus their attention too narrowly and concretely, mistakenly thinking that the event is his or her fault, which can lead to magical thinking to fill in gaps in understanding, resulting in ideas like, "if I had just been obedient, listened to my mother when she asked me to put my toys away, this war or this tsunami wouldn't have happened."[8] Often, information portrayed in the media is too complex and cognitively difficult for a young child to comprehend, particularly when the media coverage involves discussions of social and political issues. The resulting feelings of self-blame and confusion are sometimes unintentionally reinforced by adults in the child's life. When adults become stressed themselves, in the face of their displaced status, they too are more likely to become much more irritable and lose their temper. A young child may think that the adult is yelling at him or her. This situation raises the importance of developing interventions targeting parents of displaced or refugee children.

Another important developmental feature in children of this age is their inability to understand death as permanent. They often manifest their emotional responses to stressful situations with sleep difficulties such as trouble falling asleep or staying asleep and nightmares. Worry and anxiety can be manifested as clinging behavior in the form of refusing to leave the side of their adult caretaker, refusing to go to school or play, and worrying that something bad might happen to them or their parents. In addition, many may exhibit an increase in temper tantrums.[11,12]

School Age (7–11 Years)

Children at this age have acquired the ability to take other points of view and perspective. However, they remain concrete in their thinking, making many traumatic experiences difficult for them to accurately and fully comprehend. As a result, children of this age often become fearful, confused, and anxious after traumatic events. A common response is regression, or acting younger than one's age. Such regressive behaviors may include bed-wetting, thumb sucking, baby talk, and wanting to carry a transitional object like a blanket or favorite toy.[12] Children of this age may also develop physical symptoms such as loss of appetite, stomachaches, and headaches. In addition, school-related issues are common, such as impaired concentration, school refusal, or increased defiance and aggression.[13] Preoccupation with fear and danger may surface, resulting in chronic states of alarm and hyperreactivity or dissociative states.[14] School-aged children may also experience loss of interest in activities and indulge in repetitious traumatic play and retelling of the trauma.[15] Children are aware of their parents' worries most of the time but are particularly sensitive to their parents' reactions during a crisis. Looking to their parents for cues on how to act and react helps children to know how to behave in the face of danger. It is especially important for parents to be honest with their school-aged children about their fears and concerns and to stress their abilities to cope with the situation.

Teenage Years (>12 Years)

From a developmental standpoint, teenagers have developed the ability to think abstractly. With this capacity for abstract thought comes an increased focus on religion, morality, and ethics, which can affect a teenager's understanding of, and response to, acts of war and terrorism leading to their status as exiles or displaced refugees. Teenagers are also much more likely to keep their thoughts and feelings about the traumatic events inside, making them much more prone to developing depressed feelings. Teenagers may begin to withdraw from family and friends and may minimize their worries and concerns in an attempt to appear as if everything is alright.[8] In such instances, teenagers may also become increasingly irritable and defiant and may wish for revenge against the perpetrators who they feel are responsible for their current living status and undue stress. In addition, it is important to consider that those who feel particularly alienated and/or disenfranchised as a result of the painful events that they are forced to endure may be especially susceptible to the influence of terrorist organizations.

The developmental course of childhood renders the unfolding of reactions to stressful and traumatic situations a dynamic process reflecting the interplay between risk and protective factors that change with time. Some children exposed to such situations may experience immediate symptom onset, whereas others may not manifest symptoms of distress until weeks or months later.[16,17] Children who have had to face numerous losses and threats regardless of the cause of such painful events are at great risk psychologically hindering their optimal development. States of warfare, terrorism, and natural disasters including displacement affect the spectrum of contextual, interpersonal, and intrapersonal realms. Because a child's environment is multilayered, there are many factors that influence and steer a child's development such as the biology of the child itself intertwined with family, community, and societal frameworks. When any one of these layers is disrupted, it can have a ripple effect throughout the child's life.[18]

The multilayered consequences of displacement

The act of displacement itself Many victims of war, terrorism, and catastrophic natural disasters around the world find themselves displaced for short or long periods of their lives. Displaced children, who are forced into exile and have to flee from their homes, are often separated from their parents and/or live without parental supervision and care. When displacement involves crossing of national borders, children and families face additional dangers, related to being smuggled, to sexual exploitation, to experiences at armed forces check points, and witnessing parental humiliation as parents try to secure or bargain for means of safe passage. The multiple tragedies that recently occurred by sinking of boats carrying migrants and refugees attempting to reach safe shores of countries in the Mediterranean are but examples of additional horrors that children may experience during displacement.[19]

Home plays an important role in identity formation and development of children. Not only are the displaced children driven from their homes with only very few personal belongings but often have no home to return to because of the destruction and damage. Even several years later, some displaced children, and many adolescents, continue to be separated from their parents because of their educational needs that could not be met in communities of origin in which the schools were destroyed.

In addition, displaced children are faced with a whole range of other losses such as a familiar environment, routine of an educational setting, social network, and usual patterns of family life. Although refugee children sometimes show impressive resilience, particular attention should be devoted to children who had traumatic experiences immediately before displacement. These children lived without their parents or with parents who had poor coping abilities while displaced, lived in families that had accumulated several stressful experiences, or were housed in large collective refugee centers. Research has shown that the children who had poorer coping capacities and lacked supportive family environment displayed high level of stress-related symptomatology throughout the refugee period, being at special risk for the development of further psychological difficulties.[20]

Many displaced children lose their family members, close relatives, and friends, and many are orphaned. In many cases, the children directly witness the violence and death of their own family members. It is even more difficult when the family members are listed as missing for a long period, as with fathers taken as prisoners of war or unidentified bodies. In a war situation, fathers are usually called away to fight and are absent from the family for a long period.

Once relocated in a new hosting country, refugee children and families face additional problems related to seeking asylum status and the legalistic processes involved. A study from Denmark found that protracted stays and multiple relocations within the asylum system raised the odds for internalizing and externalizing symptom scores in children.[21] Postmigration living conditions contributed additional mental health risk for depression and anxiety symptoms (over and above the contribution of premigration trauma) in a sample of Burmese refugees in Australia.[22] More alarming is emerging evidence that asylum seekers with mental disorders may be less likely to be approved for asylum.[23]

Living with distressed adults Many adult members of displaced families find themselves having to endure multiple stressors and trying challenges. Often, fathers returning home at the end of the war are themselves injured and unable to find a job or able to work on account of their injuries. They feel degraded and demoralized, having to become financially dependent, and helpless. These cumulative negative effects produce high levels of stress among the adults with disturbing consequences on children. In many traditional cultures and societies, the mother is placed in a new role of being the bread winner, shifting the family hierarchy and generating conflict within families.[24,25]

This stress leads to increased family stress and marital discord and an increase in alcohol and substance use and domestic violence. Studies suggest that during warfare displaced adults frequently display anxiety, depression, anger, aggression, alcohol abuse, distrust, somatization or escape to illness, and sleep disturbance.[26]

Loss of traditional way of life Many children go through an acculturation process during which they lose contact with traditional values and ways of living in their new surroundings and communities. These losses leave a big impact on the lives of many children. Children go through another stressful and painful period of reintegration if they do return to their original towns, villages, and cities.[27,28] Spirituality and religion often serve as anchors to help both adults and children to get through difficult time. Under such circumstances, these cultural and religious practices get disrupted. In a survey done 3 to 5 days after the 9/11 events in New York City, 90% of the adults turned to religion to help cope and another 98% were helped by talking to others.[29]

Disruption of education With frequent school interruptions and decreased educational quality, teenagers have much time but few opportunities to spend it in any enjoyable or useful way. They get bored, with nothing constructive to occupy their minds and have poor coping skills. Exposed to almost daily acts of injustice, violence, and danger, negative attitudes tend to prevail, and they develop a sense of lack of purpose with hopelessness, helplessness, and demoralization. Although extensive efforts to organize schooling for all displaced children are often undertaken, less than half of the children are enrolled immediately after their arrival, in whatever educational setting is available given the circumstances. The major reason for this low level of enrollment is that many parents do not want their children to start a new school, as they hope to soon go back to their original homes. Over time, many students start to display numerous difficulties in adapting to the new educational environment, as they long for their old schools.[30]

When internally displaced or refugee children and adolescents do not return to their original homes and are not integrated into the educational system, they also fall prey to getting recruited into fundamentalist, military, or extremist groups. They end up carrying arms and engaging in combat as child soldiers, which only retraumatizes them further.[31]

Less-than-optimal physical environment Having been displaced from their homes, communities, or even countries of origin, many displaced persons are accommodated in collective centers. In many cases, 2 or even 3 families with children have to share a single room. In most such centers, there is often no place for play activities or learning. At times, families and children who come from rural areas may be accommodated in high-rise refugee centers in larger cities; not surprising, this poses major problems as to what children can do in such tight and constrained spaces when they are used to the openness of the rural communities that they come from. Even those accommodated with host families experience a lack of space. They are faced with high social density, lack of privacy, and often a poor quality of housing.[20]

Changes in the community Mass displacement whether voluntary or involuntary can lead to overwhelming distress at the community level.

These changes include the following:

- Loss of community balance and distortion of typical community value
- Increased prejudice and social rigidity toward other groups
- Problem of integration into a new social environment, emphasized in refugee and resettled families
- Changes in priorities of the social welfare, health, and educational system

Physical effects

Physical injuries leading to incapacitation and handicap The physically disfiguring injuries remain permanent reminders of the fear, horror, sadness, and pain experienced by the survivors of such injuries. The real and imagined reactions of others to their disfigured bodies present survivors with the additional and ongoing trauma of feeling rejected, isolated, unworthy, and humiliated. Millions of children eventually succumb to their injuries, whereas twice as many become physically handicapped and disabled after they have been wounded.[32] Many injured children become permanently disabled; this seriously incapacitates the child, resulting in prolonged suffering, hospitalizations, and rehabilitation.[20] Children who have been physically normal and rendered disfigured must recreate themselves, adapting their previous self-concepts and world views. Cognitively, the demand is to accommodate the altered body and new life experiences. Children must discover new ways of functioning to accomplish tasks that were once easily completed and develop new interpersonal skills as a handicapped and/or disfigured child.[33,34]

Neurodevelopmental effects

Cognition, memory, and attention Cognitive and academic impairment in traumatized youth have been consistently documented in several studies.[35,36] Language delays have been reported in abused youth.[37] Studies of preschool youth under such circumstances report significantly decreased intelligence compared with controls.[38] Being displaced can be overwhelming for anyone, but especially for a child, disrupting homeostasis and creating a compensatory response that leads to a less functional new state of equilibrium.[14] All parts of the brain are affected, cortex, limbic system, midbrain, and brainstem, with different types of traumatic memories created.[14,39–41]

Similarly, the chronic violence present in states of war and terrorism can give rise to a variety of cognitive distortions and attribution and expectancy biases. Research indicates that youth exposed to chronic violence and distress are more likely to expect violence, hostility, and aggression in their environments and to perceive these traits to exist even when they objectively do not. The hostile attribution bias, the attribution of hostile intent to others when no such intent exists, is common among individuals exposed to chronic violence.[13] In a dangerous and violent world, one can see how these mechanisms would be helpful and likely serve to protect an individual from an evil and unforgiving world. Unfortunately, however, such cognitive biases and distortions also limit the individual's capacity to see issues more broadly, allowing a person to only narrowly focus on, and sometimes even misperceive, threatening cues denying them the opportunity to attend to other environmental cues and serving to push others away.

Psychological effects

There is increasing evidence that children who are victims of trauma are prone to behavioral and emotional difficulties. Cicchetti and Toth[42] noted a wide range of effects, including affect dysregulation, disruptive and aggressive behaviors, insecure and atypical attachment patterns, impaired peer relationships with either increased aggression or social withdrawal, and academic underachievement. High rates of other comorbid psychiatric disorders, including depression, conduct disorder, attention-deficit hyperactivity disorder (ADHD), oppositional defiant disorder (ODD), and posttraumatic stress disorder (PTSD), have also been reported by the same researchers. Others have reported significant global impairment, poor social competence, major depression, conduct disorder, ODD, agoraphobia, overanxious disorder, ADHD, and substance abuse.[43–47]

Anxiety disorders and posttraumatic stress disorder Not all youth exposed to traumatic events with or without being displaced go on to develop PTSD. The stressfulness of an event depends in part on the psychobiological surface on which it strikes. Research has provided us with insight into some of the factors that likely mediate the relation between stressful events and the development of PTSD. The presentation of posttraumatic stress symptomatology, which often arises as a child begins to understand that something terrible has happened and he or she is in danger, may initiate a process of encoding and storage of implicit and/or explicit traumatic memories. These processes in children differ in several important ways from adult responses.[48] First, research indicates that children often display disorganized or agitated behavior rather than the fear, helplessness, and horror described in adults. Such disorganized behavior may manifest itself in the form of sleep disturbances, nightmares with vague content often not about the trauma itself, increased autonomic arousal, and psychosomatic complaints.[49] It is also common for traumatized children to reveal the effects of their trauma exposure through repetitive play expressing themes of abuse, flashbacks, constriction of affect, or avoidance of events associated with the abuse.[50] This traumatic play may eventually develop into more clearly defined intrusive thoughts, fears, and repeated nightmares with specific trauma content.[48] A foreshortened sense of the future, with accompanying reckless risk-taking behavior, is also common.

In a study examining refugee children in Croatia, older children reported more posttraumatic stress symptoms than younger children, with significant increases in symptoms among all ages 6 months after displacement. By maternal report, although child symptoms decreased at 12 months postdisplacement, more than half of the children were reported to still manifest at least 1 indicator of adjustment difficulty with 10% continuing to experience 5 or more symptoms. Symptom manifestations encompassed physiologic (eg, eating and sleep disturbances, increased sweating, concentration difficulties), behavioral (eg, defiance, aggression, hyperactivity, and withdrawal), and emotional (eg, fears of separation, despondency, general fearfulness, weeping, and nightmares) domains. A significant correlation was found between the number of stress symptoms manifested during the 6- and 12-month assessment, indicating that displacement was more damaging for some children than others.[20] Krystal[51] reported that Holocaust survivors frequently did not manifest PTSD symptoms until years after leaving the concentration camps.

Depression Depression, across all developmental levels, may be a consequence of trauma. Traumatized infants are prone to affective withdrawal, diminished capacity for pleasure, and a tendency to exhibit negative affect such as sadness and distress.[52] Symptoms of depression were studied in refugee children in Croatia using the Child Depression Inventory (CDI).[53] Children with high scores on the CDI were characterized both by higher rates of depression and anxiety. Scores for refugee children were significantly higher than in school children before the war. Scores did not differ, however, between the refugee children and a clinical sample of children who were treated before the war in a mental health institution for psychosomatic problems, school failure, depression, and anxiety. Moreover, 22% of refugee children compared with 18% of children from the clinical sample had a score of 18 or higher, considered to be clinically significant.[54]

A comparison of refugee children with a group of school children who had not been displaced during the war in Croatia revealed interesting findings. Although the displaced children had slightly higher scores on the CDI, there was no significant difference between the 2 groups, corroborating the findings of Zivcic.[54] Both groups showed more depressive symptoms compared with children of the same age who were assessed before the war.[20] A study done 2 years later found no significant differences between displaced children and a comparable group of nondisplaced children.

However, the overall level of depression was lower than in 1992 and close to the prewar time.[20] In the same study, at 6-month follow-up there was a significant decrease in depressive symptoms among refugee children. Correlation analyses revealed that the level of refugee children's depression was not related to the number of traumatic events but rather to the family situation, child's age, and the child's poor coping abilities during displacement, especially school difficulties. Deteriorating relations among family members, mother's poor relationship with the child since becoming a refugee, and the child's perception of rejection by the mother were significant correlates of the child's depression.

Behavioral disorders A frequent outcome of severe stress and trauma is aggression. Pathologic defense mechanisms, including identification with the aggressor, may play a role. Preschool children who have been traumatized engage in more frequent aggressive behavior than their peers[55] and more often attribute hostile intent to their peers.[56] Traumatized children have also been reported to be at risk for violent criminal behavior in adolescence[57] and adulthood.[58]

Aggressive and violent experiences provide a model for violence, teach aggression through reinforcement, inflict pain, and cause central nervous system injuries associated with impulsivity and emotional lability[59] and impaired judgment. Further, this creates a sense of being endangered and thus increases paranoid feelings and diminishes the child's capacity to recognize feelings and put them into words, not actions.

Alcohol and substance use Traumatized children are more prone to develop substance abuse. Alcohol serves to reduce anxiety, opiates trigger soothing dissociation, and stimulants such as cocaine activate dopaminergic and mesolimbic areas of the brain.[41]

MEDIATING VARIABLES AFFECTING THE PSYCHOSOCIAL WELL-BEING OF DISPLACED CHILDREN

Most experts agree that there are several mediating variables that affect how a child responds when exposed to the traumas of war and terrorism and are displaced either as refugees or in exile.

Type and Degree of Exposure

Two categories of trauma have been described by Terr.[49] Type I trauma produces typical PTSD symptoms after a one-time, sudden traumatic event. Type II trauma is the result of long-term repeated exposure to trauma, similar to what many physically abused youth experience. Type II trauma often results in an array of dysfunctional coping mechanisms such as denial and dissociation rather than symptoms characteristic of PTSD. Terr[49] also noted conduct disorder, ADHD, depression, and dissociative disorders as common conditions in children with histories of type II trauma. Pelcovitz and colleagues[50] likewise found higher prevalence of depression, conduct disorders, and ODD in their sample of physically abused youth. Children are faced with numerous losses, leading to stress and traumatization, due to war and terrorism. Several studies have shown that when a child is faced with multiple cumulative war-related stressors, especially in the absence of appropriate support from family and the community, problems with psychosocial functioning are to be expected.[60–62] These findings were corroborated in studies done in the Balkans.[20] The researchers clearly documented different sources of distress, psychological suffering, and problems of psychosocial adaptation in children exposed to war. In examining children's symptoms of distress in a wartime situation as measured by the Impact of Events Scale, Horowitz and colleagues[63] found that among the high-risk children, 39% were refugees, 35% were displaced, and 16% were from parts of the country where there were no crises. The high level of distress among this last group of children originated from indirect exposure to the war. The results of this study clearly indicated that children with varying degrees of exposure to the traumas of war were affected, although the risk was related to the level of exposure to the destruction caused by war.

Family Support

Several researchers have established a correlation between the overall number of stress reactions in a child and various aspects of family interaction. Special attention should be directed toward the adaptation of the mother to displacement and the changes in her relationship with the child. In a study done in Croatia, the number of adjustment difficulties in children correlated with the mother's posttraumatic stress reactions and decreases in maternal gentleness. There was also a significant correlation between the number of children's symptoms and separation from other members of the family. Such findings are in keeping with the research of McCallin and Fozzard[61] who reported a correlation between the intensity of psychosocial difficulties in the mother's adjustment to displacement and stress-related reactions in the children of Mozambique. In following the refugee children in Croatia, the third assessment, conducted 3 years after the second assessment, revealed that most children's stress-related symptoms had significantly decreased, coming close to prewar levels. Again, the number of stress-related symptoms significantly correlated with the mother's posttraumatic stress reaction score. These findings emphasize the significance of a stable emotional relationship between parents and children in strengthening the child's ability to cope with unfavorable circumstances.[20] There was also a moderately high significant correlation among the number of stress symptoms manifested by the child at each longitudinal assessment point. Therefore, children who manifested a higher number of difficulties after the first 6 months of displacement continued to manifest them after 12 months and even after 4 years. Exposure to chronic refugee stress likely exacerbated preexisting developmental propensities toward maladjustment in these children.[20] The importance of exposure to interpersonal family stress and family violence among war-exposed children was highlighted in 2 independent samples investigated in Lebanon. Fear of being beaten at home and witnessing quarrels between parents at home conferred higher odds ratios for the development and persistence of major depression, separation anxiety disorder, and PTSD after war than witnessing war events.[6,7] These findings taken together make it imperative to design interventions for war-exposed children and adolescents, targeting parents to promote positive parenting styles and skills. Evidence for the effectiveness of such intervention comes from a study in which evidence-based parenting practices were disseminated into resource-poor communities in the aftermath of war, finding clinically significant decreases in rates of corporal punishment, parental hostility toward their children, as well as improvement in the children's total Strengths and Difficulties Questionnaire scores.[64]

Family support is crucial to healthy development during the infant years. Gunnar[65] suggests that the security of attachment between an infant and caregiver buffers stress by downregulating the hypothalamic-pituitary-adrenal axis. When compared with insecurely attached infants, decreased cortisol levels have been found in 18-month-old children with secure attachments to their mother who were frightened by a clown.[66] Numerous studies have identified the key role of a responsive, predictable, and nurturing caregiver in the development of a healthy neurobiological stress response.[41] The environment thus regulates which synaptic connections survive,[67] possibly explaining the power of physical abuse, war, or other stressful situations in derailing attachment and developmental outcomes and of nurturance in sustaining secure attachments and healthy outcomes. Population-based studies have brought home the importance of investigating family environment and other childhood adversities in the context of exposure to traumatic events. These studies have shown that war exposure and multiple types of childhood adversities are correlated in nationally representative samples, making it imperative to investigate the impact of both types of stressors (adversities and traumatic events) when examining short- and long-term impact.[68] In investigating protective factors that mitigate against adverse outcomes of war, a recent study about resilience-promoting factors in war-exposed children revealed that one of the major protective elements against developing PTSD and internalizing and externalizing disorders is family support, characterized by parents spending more time playing with their children and supervising their homework.[69]

Child Variables

Child factors associated with poor prognosis for psychosocial adjustment include shyness or other impediments to socialization such as phobias or anxiety disorders and family interaction patterns that foster overdependence, creating a learned helplessness.[70] Individuals who make good psychosocial recoveries tend to be extroverted social risk takers with good impulse control and capacity for self-regulation who reach out to others for support. They live with a family group that places value on reciprocal support in times of need, representing high levels of family cohesion. Such well-adjusted families value and encourage individual autonomy within their group, as well as organization that facilitates function. Expressiveness of individual ideas is encouraged, and conflict is resolvable. Kagan[71,72] suggests that secure attachment patterns in infants are due more to a child's temperament rather than the environment, although he concedes that a negative environment can worsen an inhibited/anxious temperament. Finally, as the work of Lyons-Ruth and colleagues[73] and Beardslee and colleagues[74] have found, healthy infant-parent attachment promotes optimal development and protects against adverse outcomes. Such families are more likely to promote high self-esteem, good social skills, and positive adjustment in any individual, injured or otherwise. Adaptation is a process that occurs over time.

SUMMARY

There is much compelling evidence informing us that children and adolescents who are displaced are at risk for the development of multiple and sometimes protracted forms of biopsychosocial maladjustment. Full recovery often involves living through a difficult process of relearning, on physiologic, psychological, and social levels, and how to understand of the world without the constant threat of fear, hostility, and danger. It may neither be necessary nor beneficial to wait for the development of PTSD in children to be cared for more positively. There is a need to develop universal interventions targeting all war-exposed children to promote healthy coping and resilience building. Such interventions can be provided in school settings where children could learn these coping strategies like they learn other academic skills. In addition, more targeted interventions for children who develop disorders after war need to be disseminated into communities where there is no access to specialized mental health services. Most war-exposed and displaced children and adolescents reside in low- and middle-income countries where access to mental health services is not readily available. The international child mental health community must take upon itself the task of investigating and disseminating evidence for effective interventions so they can be provided when needed. Children and their mothers who learn resilience in the face of psychological trauma can become much more effective individuals in their communities.

REFERENCES

1. UNHCR (United Nations High Commission for Refugees). Available at: http://www.unhcr.org.
2. Winnicott DW. Deprivation and delinquency. London: Routledge. Publishing; 1992.
3. Milgram RM, Milgram NA. The effects of the Yom Kuppur war on the anxiety level in Israeli children. J Psychol 1976;34:107–13.
4. Milgram NA. War related stress in Israeli children and youth. In: Goldberg L, Brenitz S, editors. Handbook of stress: theoretical and clinical aspects. New York: The Free Press; 1982. p. 656–76.
5. Baker A. Psychological response of Palestinian children to environmental stress associated with military occupation. J Refug Stud 1991;4:237–47.
6. Karam EG, Fayyad J, Karam AN, et al. Outcome of depression and anxiety after war: a prospective epidemiologic study of children and adolescents. J Trauma Stress 2014;27(2):192–9.
7. Karam EG, Mneimneh ZN, Dimassi H, et al. Lifetime prevalence of mental disorders in Lebanon: first onset, treatment, and exposure to war. PLoS Med 2008; 5(4):e61.
8. Joshi P, O'Donnell DA, Cullins LM, et al. Children exposed to war and terrorism. In: Margaret MF, Silverman GB, editors. Children exposed to violence. Baltimore (MA): Paul H Brooks; 2006. p. 53–84.
9. Arroyo W, Eth S. Traumatic stress reactions and post-traumatic stress disorder (PTSD). In: Apfel R, Simon B, editors. Minefields in the heart: the mental health of children in war and communal violence. New Haven (CT): Yale University Press; 1996. p. 52–74.
10. Pynoos R, Nader K. Issues in the treatment of posttraumatic stress in children and adolescents. In: Wilson J, Raphael B, editors. International handbook of traumatic stress syndromes. New York: Plenum Press; 1993. p. 535–49.
11. Cooley-Quille M, Turner S, Beidel D. Emotional impact of children's exposure to community violence: a preliminary study. J Am Acad Child Adolesc Psychiatry 1995;34:1362–8.
12. Osofsky J. The effects of exposure to violence on young children. Am Psychol 1995;50:782–8.
13. Dodge KA. Social-cognitive mechanisms in the development of conduct disorder and depression. Annu Rev Psychol 1993;44:559–84.
14. Perry BD, Pollard R. Homeostasis, stress, trauma and adaptation – a neurodevelopmental view of childhood trauma. Child Adolesc Psychiatr Clin N Am 1998;7: 33–51.
15. James B. Handbook for treatment of attachment-trauma problems in children. New York: The Free Press; 1994.
16. Galante R, Foa D. An epidemiological study of psychic trauma and treatment effectiveness for children after a natural disaster. J Am Acad Child Adolesc Psychiatry 1986;25:357–63.

17. Terr LC. Chowchilla revisited: post-traumatic child's play. J Am Acad Child Adolesc Psychiatry 1983;20:741–60.
18. Bronfenbrenner U. Interacting systems in human development: research paradigms: present and future. In: Bolger N, Caspi A, editors. Persons in context: developmental processes. London: Cambridge University Press; 1988. p. 25–49.
19. United Nations News Center. Available at: http://www.un.org/apps/news/story.asp?NewsID=50677#.VUXiCqKJjIU. Accessed April 24, 2015.
20. Ajdukovic M, Ajdukovic D. Impact of displacement on the psychological well-being of refugee children. Int Rev Psychiatry 1998;10(3):186–95, 1.
21. Nielsen SS, Norredam M, Christiansen KL, et al. Mental health among children seeking asylum in Denmark–the effect of length of stay and number of relocations: a cross-sectional study. BMC Public Health 2008;8:293.
22. Schweitzer RD, Brough M, Vromans L, et al. Mental health of newly arrived Burmese refugees in Australia: contributions of pre-migration and post-migration experience. Aust N Z J Psychiatry 2011;45(4):299–307.
23. Tay K, Frommer N, Hunter J, et al. A mixed-method study of expert psychological evidence submitted for a cohort of asylum seekers undergoing refugee status determination in Australia. Soc Sci Med 2013;98:106–15.
24. Adjukovic M, Ajdukovic D. Psychological well-being of refugee children. Child Abuse Negl 1993;17(6):843–54.
25. Ajdukovic M. Mothers' perception of their relationship with their children during displacement: a six month follow-up. Child Abuse Rev 1996;5:34–49.
26. Moro LJ, Vidovic V. Psihicke promjene u djece i odraslih prognanika/Psychological changes in displaced children and adults. In: Klain E, editor. Ratna psihologija i psihijatrija/war psychology and psychiatry. Zagreb (Croatia): Ratni stozer Republike Hrvatske; 1992. p. 162–71.
27. Lopizic J. Neka iskustva u radu s djecom povratnicima na dubrovackom podrucju/Some experiences with repatriated children in Dubrovnik region. Paper presented at the 3rd Annual Conference of Croatian Psychologists. Bizovac, May 19–21, 1995.
28. Druzic O, Grl M, Kletecki M, et al. Meeting the needs of children in resettlement process in Hvatska Kostajnica. Proceedings of the International Conference on Trauma Recovery Training: lessons learned. Croatia: 1997. Vol. 61. p. 97–104.
29. Schuster MA, Stein BD, Jaycox LH, et al. A national survey of stress reactions after the September 11, 2001 terrorist attacks. N Engl J Med 2001;345:1507–12.
30. Dzepina M, Prebeg Z, Juresa V, et al. Suffering of Croatian school children during war. Croat Med J 1992;33:40–4.
31. Betancourt TS, Newnham EA, McBain R, et al. Post-traumatic stress symptoms among former child soldiers in Sierra Leone: follow-up study. Br J Psychiatry 2013;203(3):196–202.
32. Shaw JA. Children, adolescents and trauma. Psychiatr Q 2000;71:227–43.
33. Bordlieri JE, Solodky ML, Mikos KA. Physical attractiveness and nurses: perceptions of pediatric patients. Nurse Res 1985;34:24–6.
34. Cash TF. The psychology of physical appearance: aesthetics, attributes, and images. In: Cash TF, Pruzinsky IT, editors. Body images: development, deviance, and change. New York: Guilford Press; 1990. p. 51–79.
35. Coster WJ, Gersten MS, Beeghly M, et al. Communicative functioning in maltreated toddlers. Dev Psychol 1989;25:777–93.
36. McFadyen RG, Kitson WJ. Language comprehension and expression among adolescents who have experienced childhood physical abuse. J Child Psychol Psychiatry 1996;37:551–62.

37. Fox L, Long SH, Anglois A. Patterns of language comprehension deficit in abused and neglected children. J Speech Hear Disord 1988;53:239–44.
38. Vondra JI, Barnett DE, Cicchetti D. Self-concept, motivation, and competence among preschoolers from maltreating and comparison families. Child Abuse Negl 1990;14:525–32.
39. LeDoux J, Blakeney P, Meyer W, et al. Relationships between parental emotional states, family environment, and the behavioral adjustment of pediatric burn survivors. Burns 1998;24(5):425–32.
40. Castro-Alamancos MA, Connors BW. Short-term plasticity of a thalamocortical pathway dynamically modulated by behavioral state. Science 1996;272:274–6.
41. Phillips RG, LeDoux JE. Differential contribution of amygdala and hippocampus to cued and contextual fear conditioning. Behav Neurosci 1992;106:274–85.
42. Cicchetti D, Toth SL. A developmental psychopathology perspective on child abuse and neglect. J Am Acad Child Adolesc Psychiatry 1995;34:541–65.
43. Fisher AJ, Kramer RA, Hoven CW, et al. Psychosocial characteristics of physically abused children and adolescents. J Am Acad Child Adolesc Psychiatry 1997;36:123–9.
44. Kaplan SJ, Pelcovitz D, Salzinger S, et al. Adolescent physical abuse: risk for adolescent psychiatric disorders. Am J Psychiatry 1998;155:954–9.
45. Kaplan SJ, Pelcovitz D, Labruna V. Child and adolescent abuse and neglect research: a review of the past 10 years. Part I: physical and emotional abuse and neglect. J Am Acad Child Adolesc Psychiatry 1999;38:1214–22.
46. Livingston R, Lawson L, Jones JG. Predictors of self-reported psychopathology in children abused repeatedly by a parent. J Am Acad Child Adolesc Psychiatry 1993;32:948–53.
47. Famularo R, Kinscherff R, Fenton T. Psychiatric diagnoses of maltreated children: preliminary findings. J Am Acad Child Adolesc Psychiatry 1992;31:863–7.
48. Terr LC. Acute responses to external events and posttraumatic stress disorder. In: Lewis M, editor. Child and adolescent psychiatry: a comprehensive textbook. Baltimore (MD): Williams and Wilkins; 1996. p. 753–63.
49. Terr LC. Childhood traumas: an outline and overview. Am J Psychiatry 1991;148: 10–20.
50. Pelcovitz D, Kaplan S, Goldenberg B, et al. Post-traumatic stress disorder in physically abused adolescents. J Am Acad Child Adolesc Psychiatry 1994;33:305–12.
51. Krystal H. Massive psychic trauma. New York: International Universities Press; 1968.
52. Green AH. Physical abuse of children. In: Weiner J, editor. American Academy of Child and Adolescent Psychiatry textbook of child and adolescent psychiatry. Washington, DC: American Psychological Association; 1997. p. 17–38.
53. Kovacs M. Rating scale to assess depression in school-aged children. Acta Peadopsychiatr 1981;46:305–15.
54. Zivcic I. Emotional reactions of children to war stress in Croatia. J Am Acad Child Adolesc Psychiatry 1993;32:709–13.
55. Klimes-Dougan B, Kistner J. Physically abused preschoolers' responses to peers' distress. Dev Psychol 1990;26:599–602.
56. Dodge KA, Bates JE, Pettit GS. Mechanisms in the cycle of violence. Science 1990;250:1678–83.
57. Herrenkohl RC, Egolf BP, Herrenkohl EC. Preschool antecedents of adolescent assaultive behavior: a longitudinal study. Am J Orthop 1997;67:422–32.
58. Widom CS. Child abuse, neglect, and adult behavior. Criminology 1989;27: 251–71.

59. Lewis DO. Development of the symptom of violence. In: Lewis M, editor. Child and adolescent psychiatry: a comprehensive textbook. 3rd edition. Baltimore (MD): Lippincott Williams and Wilkins; 2002. p. 387–99.
60. Ressler EM, Boothby N, Steinbock DJ. Unaccompanied children. New York: Oxford University Press; 1988.
61. McCallin M, Fozzard S. The impact of traumatic events on the psychological well-being of Mozambican refugee women and children. Geneva (Switzerland): International Catholic Child Bureau; 1990.
62. Garbarino J, Kostelny K, Dubrow N. No place to be a child: growing up in a war zone. Lexington (MA): Lexington Books; 1991.
63. Horowitz M, Wilner N, Alvarez W. Impact of event scale: a measure of subjective stress. Psychosom Med 1979;41:209–18.
64. Fayyad JA, Farah L, Cassir Y, et al. Dissemination of an evidence-based intervention to parents of children with behavioral problems in a developing country. Eur Child Adolesc Psychiatry 2010;19(8):629–36.
65. Gunnar M. Quality of early care and buffering of neuroendocrine stress reactions: potential effects on the developing human brain. Prev Med 1998;27:208–11.
66. Nachmias M, Gunnar M, Mangelsdorf S, et al. Behavioral inhibition and stress reactivity: the moderating role of attachment security. Child Dev 1996;67:508–22.
67. Glaser D. Child abuse and neglect and the brain – a review. J Child Psychol Psychiatry 2000;41:97–116.
68. Itani L, Haddad YC, Fayyad J, et al. Childhood adversities and traumata in Lebanon: a national study. Clin Pract Epidemiol Ment Health 2014;10:116–25.
69. Fayyad J, Cordahi-Tabet C, Yeretzian J, et al. Resilience promoting factors in war exposed adolescents: an epidemiologic study, in press.
70. Blakeney P, Herndon D, Desai M, et al. Long-term psychological adjustment following burn injury. J Burn Care Rehabil 1988;9:661–5.
71. Kagan J. The nature of the child. New York: Basic Books; 1984.
72. Kagan J. Three seductive ideas. Boston: Harvard University Press; 1998.
73. Lyons-Ruth K, Connell DB, Grunebaum H. Infants at social risk: maternal depression and family support services as mediators of infant development and security of attachment. Child Dev 1990;61:85–98.
74. Beardslee WR, Salt P, Versage EM, et al. Sustaining change in parents receiving preventive interventions for families with depression. Am J Psychiatry 1997;154:510–5.

Child and Adolescent Mental Health in Haiti

Developing Long-Term Mental Health Services After the 2010 Earthquake

Rupinder K. Legha, MD[a,b,*], Martine Solages, MD[c]

KEYWORDS

• Haiti • Earthquake • Child mental health • Structural violence • Child protection

KEY POINTS

- Structural violence and the lack of child protection in Haiti assault children's well-being and their parents' ability to nurture healthy emotional and physical development. However, strong family and community ties can mitigate children's vulnerability.
- The 2010 Haiti earthquake highlighted a lack of pre-existing formal biomedical mental health services and worsened the impact of structural violence on children's well-being.
- Developing a sustainable mental health care system for children in Haiti demands a bio-psycho-social approach that capitalizes on the strengths of Haitian children, their families, and communities.
- Haiti's history of foreign aid and exploitation must inform international organization's efforts, which should be based on accompaniment and support of Haitian providers and community members.

INTRODUCTION

On January 12, 2010, a catastrophic 7.1 earthquake struck the capital of Port-au-Prince, killing 250,000 people, injuring 300,000, and displacing another 150,000, half of whom resettled in surrounding regions that were not prepared to receive them.[1] Homes, schools, churches—the structures comprising the fabric of daily

Funding Source: American Psychiatric Association, Substance Abuse and Mental Health Services Administration- Grant number, SM-11-005 (Dr R.K. Legha); None (Dr M. Solages).
Conflict of Interest: None.
[a] Dr. Mario Pagenel Fellow in Global Mental Health Service Delivery, Partners in Health, 888 Commonwealth Avenue, Boston, MA 02215, USA; [b] Program in Global Mental Health and Social Change, Department of Global Health and Social Medicine, Harvard Medical School, 641 Huntington Avenue, Boston, MA 02115, USA; [c] Department of Psychiatry and Behavioral Sciences, Children's National Medical Center, 111 Michigan Avenue, Northwest, Washington, DC 20010, USA
* Corresponding author. Partners in Health, 888 Commonwealth Avenue, Boston, MA 02215.
E-mail address: rlegha@pih.org

Child Adolesc Psychiatric Clin N Am 24 (2015) 731–749
http://dx.doi.org/10.1016/j.chc.2015.06.004 **childpsych.theclinics.com**
1056-4993/15/$ – see front matter

life—were destroyed, resulting in incomprehensible suffering in a country already rife with structural violence. In the aftermath, efforts were made to address the mental and emotional needs of children, but the scope of the disaster combined with Haiti's fragile infrastructure and limited pre-existing mental health services restricted their impact.[2] Later that spring, 2 children who had survived the earthquake and migrated to the nearby town of Mirebalais, located 60 km outside of Port-au-Prince, jumped from their school window after feeling the ground shake as a large truck drove by. Worried that another earthquake had struck, the youngsters instinctively bolted from the second story and landed on the concrete below, losing consciousness and suffering significant physical injuries. Despite a massive humanitarian effort and billions of dollars in aid, the earthquake's aftershocks continue to reverberate throughout the country. Haiti is a young country with some estimates indicating that one-third of the population is under the age of 15.[3,4] To rebuild Haiti, or to build back better, as the slogan goes, the mental well-being of the young people, the future of Haiti, must be considered; sustainable, effective interventions must be developed that capitalize on its strengths, while also addressing its challenges.

HISTORY

Haiti's oft-cited distinction as the poorest country in the Western Hemisphere[4] obfuscates the historical basis of its poverty as well as the fortitude of its poor majority. It had proud beginnings becoming the first black republic in the world in 1804 after slaves successfully overthrew their French colonial oppressors and declared independence. The "Pearl of the Antilles" had been the most lucrative French colony, contributing two-thirds of French colonial revenues between 1697 and 1804. Despite extracting Haiti's wealth through a cruel plantation economy, France demanded an indemnity of 150 million francs (roughly 3 billion dollars in today's currency) following independence to compensate slave owners for their loss of human chattel, threatening to continue warfare and economic sanctions otherwise. Forced to loan the money from France, the Haitian government entered a crushing cycle of debt that endured for 60 years, during which time it took out additional loans from other foreign powers in order to sustain itself. By 1914, 80% of Haiti's budget went toward paying back additional debts to other countries, leaving little to develop the country's infrastructure and economy during the century after independence.[5]

Having abolished slavery decades before the United States and other surrounding countries, Haiti represented a significant threat to the colonial world order. As a result, outside forces strove to subjugate it politically and economically. In 1915, the US Marines landed in Haiti reportedly to bring order following a bloody coup and occupied the country for the next 2 decades. Under the pretext of democratizing Haiti's political institutions and building schools and roads, they ushered in agricultural companies who forced Haitian peasants off their land and created new plantations to advance US economic gains. To quell popular resistance, they installed a police unit that served as the predecessors to the Duvalier regime's infamous Tonton Macoute, a paramilitary force that engaged in violence and egregious human rights abuses from the 1950s through the 1980s.[6]

However, Haiti's colonial and postcolonial history fostered strengths. Branded with their masters' initials and killed by overwork and disease, slaves remarkably developed their own language and culture to sustain their African heritage. African religious practice was actively suppressed, and slaves were forced to convert to Christianity. So, over time, they developed Voudou, a hybrid form of worship that allowed them to mix various heritages and disguise outlawed cultural practices. Kreyol was also developed through a melding of different dialects, including French and other African languages. Both facilitated the personal connections that gave rise to the communities of trust and resistance that ignited the slave revolt in 1791 and paved the way for independence in 1804. Both inform contemporary Haitian culture and experience today.[6] After independence, freed slaves, who comprised the bulk of the population, lobbied for dividing the former plantations into smaller plots for them to work independently and autonomously. The elite, however, whose wealth depended on forced labor and who controlled the government, maintained the model, resulting in a 2-caste society. The vast gulf between the two—the literate, French-speaking, wealthy few, and the illiterate, Kreyol-speaking, rural poor majority—has endured for more than 200 years, and many have argued that this inequality is deliberate, intended to protect the former through an ongoing war waged against the poor.[7]

POVERTY, VIOLENCE, AND STRUCTURAL VIOLENCE

Ranked 162 of 187 countries on the Human Development Index, Haiti's gross national income per capita was $1070 in 2012, having decreased by 41% since 1980. More than 50% of Haitians live in extreme poverty, earning less than a dollar a day.[8] The unemployment rate reaches 49% in metropolitan areas and 36% in rural areas.[9] Just 1% of the population controls more than half the wealth, and 5% of the population controls 75% of arable land. Thus, the same 2-caste society that emerged after independence endures, as the country remains dominated by a small group of wealthy elite surrounded by countless destitute poor.[7] Because of deforestation for business and charcoal (90% of households rely on it for fuel), two-thirds of Haiti's once fertile land is now unsuitable for cultivation. Most Haitians, who live in the countryside and farm small plots of land for food, face significant difficulty generating enough food.[10] Domestic production of rice, the staple of the Haitian diet, has been undercut by the vast amounts of "free" American rice dumped through foreign aid.[7] As a result, farming activities have slowed, pushing peasants to leave rural areas for cities where unemployment rates have been high, shifting consumption from locally produced to imported food, which now accounts for 50% of food consumption.[11] Deforestation has also made Haiti vulnerable to floods and hurricanes, and during the 2008 season, nearly 70% of crops were destroyed, causing many children to die of malnutrition. One-third of households surveyed for a 2009 study reported economic deterioration in the prior 2 years, due to high international food prices and a deadly 2008 hurricane system.[12] Thus, numerous factors operating on multiple levels—including international efforts and natural disasters—collide to push the poor further into poverty.

Multiple other aspects of daily living are deficient. Half of all families do not have a purified water source, whereas three-fourths do not have a method of sanitized waste removal; only 25% have access to electricity services.[12,13] Transportation is difficult, because there are few paved roads and no formal public transportation system, leaving individuals to travel hours by foot to access work, school, or health care facilities.[14,15] The public sector, weakened by poor leadership and widespread corruption and undermined by international interference, lacks the means and, arguably, the will to intervene on the majority's behalf.[6] Currently, 70% of Haiti's operating budget derives from foreign aid and investment, and more than 10,000 nongovernmental organizations (NGOs) operate within Haiti, the majority without any regulation or oversight from the government.[7] The aid apparatus in Haiti, known as "The Republic of NGOs," has failed to coordinate efforts, collaborate with the public sector, and effectively manage funds. Wrought with fraud, greed, and corruption, it is often used to advance financial and political agendas, rather than the well-being of the Haitian people.[7,16]

Haiti's poverty, infrastructure, and limited opportunities make daily life harsh and rife with countless challenges; as a result, many Haitians who can leave do: almost 80% of college graduates immigrate to other countries to seek better opportunities.[17] In contrast, the poor majority, who cannot leave, live in a world of permanent insecurity, on the edge of survival with nothing to fall back on. This insecurity is based not only in poverty but also in widespread violence and repression dating back to the Duvalier dictatorship (1957–1986).[18,19] In the 22 months following the 2004 overthrow of Haiti's first democratically elected president, Jean-Bertrand Aristide, an estimated 8000 people were murdered and 35,000 women were sexually assaulted, half of whom were under the age of 18 years.[3] From 2007 to 2012, Haiti's homicide rate doubled, much of it driven by high levels of violence and gang activity in Port-au-Prince, where 75% of homicides occurred. Almost 15% of all homicides stemmed from domestic violence (63,600), the vast majority of victims being women.[20] Capturing the pervasiveness of uncertainty and danger, one survey found that three-quarters of youth ages 10 to 24 felt that most people cannot be trusted; nearly two-thirds were afraid to visit their neighbors, and half were afraid to go to the local market.[12]

CHILD PROTECTION

Children in Haiti face daily assaults to their emotional and physical well-being due to structural violence; there are few governmental/bureaucratic structures in place to protect them. Education is, perhaps, the most revealing example. Only 60% of children between ages 6 to 11 are enrolled in school; while 3 of 4 children in urban areas start primary school, only half of children in rural areas do. There is no functional public education system: more than 90% of schools are nonpublic, and most receive no state support or oversight/regulation. Families are left to finance private institutions' school fees, which average 100 dollars per year for primary school. These school fees, along with expenses for school materials and examinations, are a prohibitive factor for impoverished families on the brink; as a result, they enroll one child at a time or rotate children to give each an opportunity or withdraw children from school altogether. Class promotion, teacher qualifications, and schools fees are unregulated by the Ministry of Education, resulting in low-quality and economic exploitation, particularly of poor families desperate to educate their children. A patronage system in which school admission is brokered through social connections further interferes with access to quality education. Resources are very limited with more than half of schools lacking electricity and two-thirds without libraries. The best schools tend to be private and concentrated in the wealthiest parts of Port-au-Prince, reflecting the enduring divide between the urban elite and rural poor. Students, especially in rural areas, often leave school because of its poor quality, the need to support the family through work, or the lack of finances. The resulting high rates of repetition further increase school costs and create an education investment trap where the poorest households get no return on the money they invest in educating their children, becoming even poorer and further discouraging enrollment in school.[15]

Many parents make the difficult decision to send their children elsewhere with the hope of finding better opportunities, only to render them more vulnerable. Orphanages, which carry the promise of school, shelter, and food, are one option: roughly 80% of the 30,000 children in Haitian institutions are thought to have parents.[21] Despite their promise, most orphanages are unaccredited, and many are negligent in their care of children, some of whom are malnourished, physically and sexually abused, and at higher risk for infections.[21–23] *Restavèk*, Haitan Kreyol for "to stay with," refers to the system of sending children, usually from poor rural families, to live with relatives and strangers, and it affects approximately 200,000 (or 1 in 15) children.[24] A popular Haitian folk tale, *Ti Sentaniz*, tells the story of the title character, a 9-year-old girl, orphaned after her mother dies, sent to live with a wealthier family with the hope of receiving education, food, and shelter. Instead, she is treated like a slave, forced to rise before and go to sleep after the family to tend to an unending list of chores. Barefoot with no shoes and clad in a dress so worn her ribs are visible, 9-year-old Ti Sentaniz accompanies 14-year-old Chantoutou to school but does not attend herself. While Chantoutou sleeps in a regal bed, Sentaniz sleeps on the hard floor on a thin mat; one night Chantoutou's brother rapes her.[25] Reports from former *restavèk* indicate that the tale is not far from the truth, because they are often overworked, abused, malnourished, and denied contact with their families so much that the *restavèk* phenomenon in Haiti has been called modern-day slavery.[26–28] The family taking in the child is often only marginally better off than the family sending the child. Lacking resources to support another child, the accepting family, therefore, puts the *restavèk* child to work rather than sending him or her to school.[24]

Within the Haitian government, there have been several promising efforts to improve child protection. The Institute de Bien Etre Social et de Recherches (IBESR), a substructure within the Ministry of Social Affairs, is charged with overseeing the adoption process as well as orphanages. In 2012, with support from the United Nations Children's Fund (UNICEF), it reviewed more than 700 orphanages and ordered the closing of 72 of them due to poor quality, and it has supported efforts to reunite children with their families. The Brigade de Protection de Mineurs (BPM), a division within the Haitian National Police and also supported by UNICEF, stopped 1437 children from illegally crossing the border into the Dominican Republic from May to December 2010. Various other mandates to protect children's well-being are written, but in practice, much is left to be realized. Haiti is party to the Universal Declaration on Human Rights and the Convention on the Rights of the Child. It has also ratified International Labor Organization Conventions prohibiting child slavery and servitude, demanding children's right to education, and asserting their right to freedom from degrading and inhumane treatment. In accordance with these international conventions, Article 335 of the Haitian labor code prohibits the employment of minors less than the age of 15. Furthermore, an act passed in June 2003 specifically outlawed the placement of children into *restavèk* service and the abuse and maltreatment of children generally.[29] Despite the enactment of these laws, the practice of *restavèk* persists openly, while the school system—public and private—remains in tremendous need of oversight from the Ministry of Education.

COMMUNITY AND FAMILY

The resistance and passionate refusal of slavery that defeated the French and made Haiti the first black republic endure to the present day through an unceasing emphasis on independence and personal freedom brokered through a reliance on family and community rather than the state. Despite the postindependent government's plantation model of agriculture, peasant farmers—former slaves—managed to access small plots of land through purchase, squatting on privately owned or state-owned land, or through the *metyage* system, in which small parcels of land were leased for exchange of crops. Beyond just taking control of land, peasants developed a set of social and cultural practices intended to secure ownership and prevent reinstatement of the plantation model. The *lakou* system refers to a group of houses usually owned by an extended family gathered around a common yard. Each individual or nuclear family owns their own land, providing basic necessities for themselves, while the larger community oversees issues like inheritance and land ownership—preventing, for example, the selling of land outside of the *lakou* to avoid the acquisition of land by outside parties.[6] Closely related to the *lakou* system, the *konbit* system evolved as a way for Haitian peasants to acquire field labor through community ties, rather than payment. Peasants from the same *lakou* work their land together, rotating through every family's plot during the harvest time. Each individual participant is fed by the family whose plot is tilled, and eventually all plots of land are properly harvested.

Although the *lakou* and *konbit* systems evolved after independence, they prevail even today; although rooted in rural life, versions have been transplanted into urban settings like Port-au-Prince too and even within the diaspora. Children are raised not only by their families but also within the extensive familial and social networks. Solidarity exists within communities such that if one family does not have enough food to eat, for example, another family will share what it has, or if one family is facing a conflict or loss, other members of the community will contribute by sharing resources or participating in decision-making. Families may even send a child to live with other family or friends if their economic situation worsens and they are unable to provide. What families may lack individually due to poverty, they strive to overcome through social connection, which, in turn, can create a powerful safety net. Haitians also take pride in trusting that they have the inner strength to cope with most challenges, a resolve bolstered by religious and spiritual faith, including the practice of Voudou.[30] All of these adaptive social enterprises, grounded in Haiti's origins and historical bravery, have endured in part because of the state's inability to protect its poor rural majority from structural violence.[6]

Communities reinforce the existing family structure, for which *fanm se poto mitan* or women are the center post.[31] Mothers are held primarily responsible for their children, but in rural areas, they may also work the land or engage in small business ventures, like street-side stands. Fathers are charged with being providers and protectors, ensuring safety, security, and the provision of basic necessities. Children are thought to be gifts from God, and parents (specifically mothers) will do almost anything to ensure that their children's basic needs are met, even if it means neglecting their own basic needs. Respect for elders is emphasized, and children are generally raised to be well-behaved, obedient, and deferential to authority figures. Unfortunately, a growing proportion of children in Haiti are growing up in single-parent households. One survey found that only half of youth (10–24) were living with both parents, and 1 of 5 had lost both because of abandonment or illness.[12] Sometimes these children are absorbed into extended family networks, but they become very vulnerable when these safety nets are not available.

HEALTH CONTEXT PRE-EARTHQUAKE

Maternal and Child Health

Haiti's poverty, structural violence, and limited infrastructure collide, negatively impacting their physical health and well-being even before birth. Most Haitian women deliver their babies at home without a skilled attendant present; although 80% of women have at least one prenatal visit, this does not necessarily ensure sufficient education, vaccinations, or instruction about potential complications.[32] Financial constraints and physical distance, which limit access to care, along with few treatment resources contribute to high rates of infections, including syphilis, which carries a high infant fatality rate.[33–35] Four of 10 women are the victims of violence during pregnancy, mainly interpersonal violence.[36] Capturing the cumulative impact of these health inequities, the maternal mortality in 2008 was 630 per 100,000 women (compared with 63 per 100,000 women across the Americas), with eclampsia, hemorrhage, and infection, all of which are potentially treatable, as the main causes of death. Although infant and child mortalities have declined markedly in the last few decades, they remain significantly higher than other countries in the Western hemisphere and are worse in rural areas. Child death is so common that mothers sometimes wait several years to name their children, and there are countless mothers who have watched all of their children precede them in death. According to the Pan American Health Organization (PAHO)/World Health Organization (WHO), the main causes of infant death in Haiti include acute diarrheal disease, intestinal infectious diseases, infections of the perinatal period, malnutrition, and acute respiratory infections. In schoolchildren, common causes of death include infectious and parasitic diseases, and among adolescents, the main causes of death are HIV/AIDS, assault, homicide, tuberculosis and typhoid.[37] The prevalence of HIV has declined since the 1990s, due to combined efforts by the ministry of health and various NGOs, but less than half of pregnant women receive HIV counseling and testing, with access being more limited in rural areas.[38] Among children with respiratory illnesses, less than 10% receive antibiotics. Furthermore, the overall immunization rate of children less than 2 years of age was 41% 2 years before the earthquake. Chronic malnutrition effects 22.2% of children under the age of 5; acute, severe malnourishment, 4.3% of children; and the vast majority of children ages 6 to 59 months have anemia.[39,40] These various statistics must be understood in terms of the structural violence—the poor sanitation and hygiene, food and water insecurity, and poor health care infrastructure—that underlie them.

Child Neurodevelopmental and Mental Health

There are limited data about child mental health and neurologic disorders in Haiti, but some conclusions can be extrapolated. Abuse and neglect are thought to be common: one survey sample found that 60% of adult women and 85% of men had experienced abuse or neglect as children.[41] Studies of Haitian immigrant youth have noted extensive trauma in a variety of different contexts, including witness to political killings and torture and abuse by stepparents, as well as high rates of depression and posttraumatic stress disorder (PTSD).[42,43] Working as a *restavek*; exposure to gang, political, and street violence; and leaving Haiti to work in the Dominican Republic, where mistreatment and abuse are common, almost certainly predispose children and adolescents to trauma and emotional distress.[44,45] Any separation from the safety net of family and community, including being sent to an orphanage or to another family/friend where school or basic needs are more available, could predispose youth to abuse and neglect. Poverty, of course, drives all of these phenomena, which tend to be interrelated. A 2005 survey of more than 20,000 homes in Haiti found that one-third had orphaned and vulnerable children. Among this subgroup, nearly one-half were exposed to male-perpetrated physical or sexual violence against female intimate partners in the preceding year, and they were more likely to live with an HIV-infected parent than nonorphaned and vulnerable children.[46] Thus, structural violence in all its forms assaults the development and well-being of children in Haiti.

Children of parents with HIV/AIDS endure stigma and discrimination, resulting in anxiety and symptoms of depression.[47,48] Close to one-fifth of young women are sexually assaulted but lack judicial recourse against their perpetrators and often have their or their family members' lives threatened if they disclose.[49] Lack of education and unemployment, which disproportionately plague the poor, can negatively shape life prospects and visions for the future, while lacking social support and family support, due to parental death or family conflict, can predispose Haitian youth to emotional distress and mental illness.[15,43,45,47] The high burden of psychological distress among the adult population, many of whom are parents, unquestionably impacts the adjustment and emotional health of their children.[41,50] Estimates of neurodevelopmental disabilities and disorders, such as epilepsy and intellectual disabilities, are unavailable, but the high rates of neonatal infections, birth injuries, and malnutrition that impact children in other low income countries have very likely resulted in disproportionately high prevalence in Haiti, too.[51] Children with cognitive and physical disabilities are at risk for abandonment and exploitation, and many children with physical and cognitive disabilities in Haiti, including epilepsy, do not attend school. The cases in **Boxes 1** and **2** underscore how bio-psycho-social risk and protective factors come together to create complex clinical presentations and challenging treatment dilemmas for children and their families.

Health Care System

Haitian children and their families contend with these formidable health care challenges in the context of a fragmented, threadbare, and oversubscribed biomedical health care services, which are described in greater detail in a 2011 document

Box 1
Case 1

A 7-month-old baby is brought to a nearby hospital in rural Haiti and treated for a skull fracture after her 18-year-old mother held her by the feet and hit her head against the ground for reasons that are not clear. The baby, who is otherwise well-nourished and healthy, suffers no major sequelae, but a hospital psychologist, one of few in the country, is consulted to determine whether the baby's mother is mentally ill. The family lives in a rural area that is only accessible by boat and foot, making travel to and from the hospital difficult. Therefore, the psychologist seeks to develop an alliance with the baby's maternal grandmother and arranges for a home visit to meet the mother when the baby is discharged.

Upon arriving in the family's village, neighbors and extended family congregate at the baby's home, relieved that she has returned safely. After finding a secluded area to meet with the 18-year-old mother, the psychologist learns that she has been severely depressed, weighed down by the responsibilities of caring for a baby. Following an argument in which her mother asked her to leave home, she tried to kill the baby and had planned to kill herself by slitting her neck with a machete, but she was instead tied up by members of the local village, some of whom threatened to harm her. She has been raising the baby without any emotional or financial support from the baby's father and, as her own mother's oldest child, feels significant guilt for burdening her mother so heavily. Shortly after her own birth, her father abandoned her and her mother, both of whom suffered financial hardship as a result. The baby, mother, and grandmother live in a simple one-room structure made of cement and farm a small plot of land for food and commerce, although their economic situation is precarious. The mother, who has never attended school, aborted a baby several years earlier after a neighbor raped and impregnated her. It is not clear whether sex was brokered for financial support from this neighbor.

The psychologist's visit centers around evaluating and supporting the 18-year-old mother, ensuring her and her baby's safety, providing psycho-education to family and neighbors, and strengthening the alliance with the baby's grandmother. In particular, he notes how the mother's severe depression and trauma history led to her actions and explains the need for ongoing treatment. The grandmother agrees to let the mother move back home and assumes primary responsibility for the baby, along with several other family members living in the same village. The psychologist works with a supportive aunt and local leader who agree to visit the mother daily to ensure her well-being. Transportation is arranged for a follow-up visit at the local hospital the following week to continue mental health care and to complete a full medical evaluation.

Box 2
Case 2

A 9-year-old girl is evaluated at a local clinic in rural Haiti for a presumptive diagnosis of epilepsy. Several weeks earlier, the girl was treated at the same clinic for a diarrheal illness; during that visit, a clinic physician began antiepileptic medication. The seizures, which began at age 7 and had never been treated, have decreased in frequency. A psychologist meets with the girl and her mother to conduct a comprehensive mental health evaluation and to address the psychosocial dimensions of epilepsy. During the evaluation, the mother reports that her daughter sustained physical trauma during birth and was slow to meet major milestones, including talking and advancing in school, especially relative to her cousins of the same age. Throughout the meeting, the mother is very attentive to her daughter, straightening her dress and encouraging her to speak politely with the psychologist. The girl, who is pleasant and cheerful, draws a picture of herself smiling and wearing a red dress. Its lack of complexity suggests that her development has been slowed.

The mother, clearly invested in her daughter's care, nonetheless appears sad. She eventually confesses her concern about ongoing possession by a spirit, which she believes is the cause of her daughter's *kriz* (seizure). Visits to a local traditional healer and prayer at church were unsuccessful at eliminating the *kriz*. Therefore, the mother heeded family members' advice to remove her from school and sent her to a faraway village to stay with other family members in order to escape the spirit. As a result, the mother and daughter have been separated from one another for several months. The mother runs a small food stand to earn a limited income, while her husband works a small plot of land in order to feed them and their 5 children. Because of her financial limitations and responsibility to her other young children, she has not been able to visit her daughter regularly. Having always sensed that her daughter is more vulnerable, the mother worries because she does not attend school and is not closely supervised. She eventually bursts into tears while her daughter, worried, sits next to her holding her hand and looking down.

While another clinician takes the girl for a walk, the psychologist meets with the mother privately and asks more detailed questions about her daughter's safety and well-being, including whether she is being mistreated or abused in her new home. He validates the mother's worries and supports her dedication to her daughter. He provides extensive psycho-education about epilepsy, including its cause, and normalizes the mother's belief system by noting that many people in Haiti believe that this devastating illness is caused by possession of a spirit. He also strongly recommends reuniting the daughter with her family and sending her back to school. He and the mother agree to meet again without the daughter present in order to discuss the epilepsy and developmental disorder, and to evaluate the mother for depression. The daughter is evaluated by a pediatrician and is found to be in good health with no signs of abuse or neglect. A community health worker is asked to meet with the mother at home to provide more information about epilepsy and to discuss associated stigma related to misconceptions of the illness. The mother leaves feeling more hopeful and reassured about her daughter's well-being.

published by the WHO and the PAHO.[52] Almost one-half of the population of Haiti has no access to formal health care services. Only 30% of health care facilities are public, operated by the Ministry of Health (Ministère de la Santé Publique et de la Population, MSPP), and most of them are in urban areas. They are unequipped and undersupplied in part because health care expenditures only account for 7% of the government's total budget. In rural areas, 70% of health services are provided by NGOs and include mainly primary health care. Health care resources are very limited and highly centralized, and there is no network of care or referral system. Nearly 90% of all Haitian physicians practice in just one geographic locale, the West Department (which includes the capital city of Port-au-Prince).[9]

Mental health care, which comprises only 1% of the already insufficient health care budget, has historically centered around 2 psychiatric facilities in Port-au-Prince. Mars and Klein and Beudet, which have an inpatient capacity of 140 to 200 adults, were in a broken-down state even before the earthquake, too poorly financed and staffed to provide quality care.[2,53,54] Three other private centers (with 100 beds in total) and psychological units in 2 private hospitals in Port-au-Prince offer psychological and psychiatric services to affluent members of the community. In other regions of Haiti, four units in public hospitals (all in urban settings) provide basic services, such as assessment and support, led by 1 or 2 psychologists and 2 or 3 nurses.[54] To the authors' knowledge, none of these facilities provide specialized, dedicated care for children, and there are no neurologists in Haiti, either. In 2003, there were just 10 psychiatrists, none of whom were trained child psychiatrists, and 9 psychiatric nurses working in Haiti's public sector, primarily in Port-au-Prince.[9,52] Access to mental health in rural areas, where 60% of the population resides, is severely limited, and there is no national mental health plan or strategy and no national formularies or treatment guidelines for care.[2] Furthermore, there is no apparatus in place for early identification of and intervention for developmental delays, and special education services are virtually nonexistent.

Beliefs and Values Related to Mental and Neurologic Illness

In 2011, WHO and PAHO published a literature review of culture and mental health in Haiti, and it provides a useful overview of how religion, spirituality, and other value systems shape perceptions of mental illness.[9] Illness is often viewed as being brought on either by God (*maladi bondye*) or by magic (*maladi maji*), which is thought of as someone, such a jealous neighbor or offended spirit (*lwa*), cursing the patient and causing the illness.[55] Epileptic seizures, in particular, are construed as evidence of spirit possession.[56,57] Voudou, based on worship and possession of the spirits, is practiced extensively throughout Haiti, although individuals often concurrently practice other religions, particularly Catholicism, the predominant religion in Haiti, but increasingly Protestantism and other Christian-based faiths.[9] These explanatory models inform treatment-seeking patterns because individuals almost always seek services from priests, clergymen, or Voudou priests before considering biomedical care.[58]

In terms of emotional distress and mental illness, these explanatory models apply with several additional caveats. Because of the interconnectedness and reliability of families and communities, individuals will often pursue advice or help from social networks before advancing to religious or spiritual outlets, maybe never pursuing biomedical care at all.[59] Depression may be somaticized, leading to presentation in primary care clinics, and idioms of distress are often used to convey symptoms.[60] For example, *pedi bon sans li* (losing one's good senses) often signifies psychosis, while *kè sere* (heartbreak) suggests anxiety, and *maladi tonbè* (falling sickness) can refer to possible seizure.[61] Spiritual, religious, familial, and community outlets can be protective, but stigma, discrimination, and mistreatment can result: people suffering from mental illness can be ostracized, beaten, tied up, or locked up. As a result, by the time they arrive at a mental health clinic, their situation is likely to be more urgent. Explanatory models are not mutually exclusive, and individuals often pursue biomedical care as they seek spiritual and religious outlets, too.[9] Although explanatory models are important, structural factors, specifically the unavailability of biomedical treatment and the scarcity of skilled providers, dictate care seeking and the resulting treatment gap for mental and neurologic illness.[62] It is perhaps not surprising that widespread, devastating illnesses, like HIV/AIDS and epilepsy, have been construed as the consequence of outside forces beyond the individual's control, given that people often end up burned and maimed in the case of epilepsy or dead in the case of both because treatment is unavailable or inaccessible. It is also not surprising that Haitians, particularly the rural poor, use whichever resources are at their disposal in order to make sense of their reality and survive it, as they have done this since their country's inception.

AFTER THE EARTHQUAKE MENTAL HEALTH NEEDS

In the aftermath of the earthquake, nearly 300,000 homes and 4000 schools, or 80% of the schools in Port-au-Prince, were badly damaged or destroyed;600,000 individuals left their homes, and up to 1.5 million people ended up residing in internally displaced camps (IDPs).[63] In addition to the immediate shock and trauma, survivors, including children, suffered additional stress because they were unable to save the trapped and help the injured. Rescue tools were unavailable, health facilities were overwhelmed, first aid capacity was limited, and many roads were blocked. In some cases, victims were surrounded by corpses for several days, until the authorities were able to clear them.[64] Children's physical traumas ranged from minor scrapes and bruises to debilitating orthopedic injuries and burns, unilateral or bilateral amputations, and severe facial and skull fractures, which were treated in makeshift field hospitals erected amid the rubble. Many children received medical care alone.[65,66] All of the pre-existing challenges related to structural violence, limited public sector capacity, and health inequity exploded, resulting in even greater challenges related to children's basic needs, safety, and protection. Parents died and families were fractured as the injured were rushed to health care facilities. There were no systematic efforts to record, identify, and trace children who were lost, and unaccompanied children requiring medical care were sometimes discharged to the street or kept inpatient indefinitely.[21] Risks for child trafficking soared because there was no system for identifying legitimate institutional facilities and protecting children against abduction. One American church group attempted to abduct 33 children with the hopes of moving them to an orphanage in the Dominican Republic, even though all of them had at least one living parent.[67] Children without parents were particularly vulnerable in the IDP camps, where sexual assaults of girls and women were common.[68,69]

In total, 750,000 children were directly or indirectly affected; 30,000 children were displaced, and 9000 children were officially registered with UNICEF as "separated" from their families, although the numbers are thought to be higher.[70] Exact estimates of rape victims were not available, but a March 2010 survey estimated that 3% of all people in Port-au-Prince had been sexually assaulted, almost entirely women with half of the victims less than age 18.[68] The government reported that at least 150,000 corpses were buried in mass graves, preventing proper burials and appropriate grieving in accordance with Haitian religious and spiritual values.[2,71] Economic hardships following the earthquake led to an increase in the number of children whose families sent them to out-of-home care, and up to 1 of 5 families in Haiti's Central Plateau took in someone displaced by the earthquake. Parents lost their work, while children lost their schooling, and both lost the routines and structures of their daily lives. An October 2010 cholera outbreak traced to a United Nations battalion from Nepal resulted in 200,000 infections and 6000 deaths in the following 9 months and complicated matters further.[63] There were no widespread efforts to quantify the unimaginable distress and mental health sequelae among children and adolescents, although exceedingly high rates of PTSD (37%) and clinical depression (46%) have been documented in school-aged children impacted by the earthquake.[72] Those with traumatic physical injuries may have suffered additionally from stigma and exclusion from school. Children who were vulnerable before the earthquake, due to being *restavek*, living in orphanages, suffering from extreme poverty or abuse, or being separated from family, were undoubtedly rendered even more defenseless.

AFTER THE EARTHQUAKE MENTAL HEALTH RESPONSE

During the weeks following the earthquake, NGOs and local mental health clinicians performed psychosocial assistance activities and mental health services. The Haitian government under MSPP attempted to organize efforts through the United Nations Cluster approach in accordance with the Sphere Standards and the recommendations of the Inter-Agency Standing Committee (IASC). IASC guidelines centered on the imperative to do no harm and to provide varying levels of intervention that matched the acuity of needs in different sectors of the population. These and other extensive details regarding the general mental health response have been documented elsewhere.[2] Guidelines specifically for children cautioned against pathologizing the normal, expected physiologic and emotional response to the earthquake, such as regression, and emphasized the importance of keeping children embedded within their families. Providing basic services and security, including food, shelter, livelihood, protection, and health care, the school was emphasized as the setting and foundation for all interventions, while family and community support was encouraged as a next step in the IASC pyramid approach to care. Creating safe spaces for play, bolstering community support, and developing daily routines were particularly important for children. Although psychological first aid was recommended, IASC guidelines specified that specialty psychological and psychiatric services be limited to individuals who developed severe mental disorders and vulnerable children, specifically those with neuropsychiatric disorders, including epilepsy, developmental disorders, or mental retardation, as well as children in institutional care.[64,73]

Within 6 months, the United Nations reported that emergency shelters had been distributed to more than 1.5 million people and food to 4.3 million people, and more than 1 million people had access to potable water as a result of humanitarian aid efforts. An estimated 80% of affected schools were reopened, and 55,000 children were reached through 200 child-friendly spaces.[74] Through UNICEF, 4948 children separated from their families were registered and 1265 were reunited. Of note, 40% of these cases were separated from families before the earthquake.[70] Several international agencies made efforts to prevent gender-based violence by increasing safety and building child protection capacity within the local police as well as providing legal support. However, the vast majority of victims did not receive justice or even medical treatment.[39,68,69] Within MSPP, a Haitian national mental health authority was appointed to coordinate government activities on policy, mental health legislation, and the planning of services as well as to direct the cluster. WHO and PAHO engaged in a role of support to the government and this authority, with the aim of advising on mental health policy, assisting in planning and coordination of responses, monitoring the quality of outside technical assistance, and helping to assist with reconstruction to build a sustainable national mental health service capacity and resource mobilization.[2]

Much enthusiasm followed the initial wave of earthquake response efforts. The earthquake had revealed Haiti's pre-existing vulnerabilities to an international audience eager to support it; many called on efforts to "Build Back Better"—to reconstruct and rebuild Haiti to protect it against future devastation. Unfortunately, this effort has largely failed.[75] Billions of dollars in aid were promised but never made it to Haiti or were never used. Political and bureaucratic obstacles slowed the disbursement of funds and caused disagreement about which recovery efforts to prioritize. Of the $2.43 billion in aid disbursed in 2010, only 1% went to the Haitian government; the rest went to organizations based in donor countries and the United Nations. Substantial recovery funds were dedicated to acute needs and consumable goods (food, temporary shelters, short-term jobs, water purification) rather than infrastructure, including permanent housing; the Interim Haiti Recovery Commission, an interagency group led jointly by former US President Bill Clinton and members of the Haitian Government, struggled to reach its goal and ultimately disbanded.[1] Aid and donor agencies worked around the public sector rather than with it; ordinary Haitians were left out of the rebuilding process. Four years after the earthquake, 145,000 individuals remained in the camps, 60,000 of whom were children.[2]

TOWARD LONG-TERM SUSTAINABLE SOLUTIONS FOR CHILDREN'S MENTAL HEALTH IN HAITI

Acute on chronic is a fitting analogy for the earthquake, because it was an urgent crisis occurring in the context of persistent social dysfunction, the chronic conditions amplifying the acute ones and requiring primary treatment themselves if the country is to recover. This analogy can also be extended to child mental health and well-being in Haiti. Beyond stabilizing the acute child mental health problems after the earthquake, comprehensive and sustainable interventions are needed to treat the chronic ones that underlie them. Furthermore, the mistakes characterizing the failure to build back better—and Haiti's larger history—cannot be repeated.

A national planning process is needed to guide the development of credible, scalable models of community-based child mental health care that are appropriate for the Haitian context and capitalize on its strengths. Haitian health workers and MSPP must take the lead; international players should support their efforts rather than operate around them or undermine them. Structural violence rooted in the country's history assaults children's physical and emotional well-being, and a weakened public sector cannot provide the formal child protection to offset this, resulting in devastating consequences. However, strong families and communities can offset children's vulnerability; therefore, clinical interventions must strive to keep children embedded within them. The larger sociopolitical sphere warrants strong consideration when considering child protection. Child trafficking and *restavèk*, for example, will not be eliminated until the larger social and structural factors—including the absence of a functioning public education system and economic opportunities—are rendered obsolete. Public sector institutions, such as IBESR and BPM, also need support and strengthening to ensure adequate child protection and defense of human rights. Effective clinical care requires a bio-psycho-social assessment that weighs the risk and protective factors operating on multiple levels, from the individual to the larger society that shapes children's mental health and well-being (**Table 1**). Risk factors must be mitigated, whereas protective factors should be capitalized on to provide effective clinical care, as demonstrated in the cases in **Boxes 1** and **2**. **Box 3** provides guiding principles for developing interventions to support and sustain child mental health in Haiti.

Several innovative projects have shown promise. Zanmi Lasante (ZL) Mental Health Team, in conjunction with Partners in Health, is currently implementing a pilot model of community-based mental health care in rural Haiti. Through screening tools, illness-based care pathways, and curriculum development; data-driven quality improvement and supervision; monitoring and evaluation; and the establishment of culturally appropriate clinical tools, standards, and guidelines, this effort is developing a system of mental health care for children and adults. Preliminary data demonstrate the feasibility of integrating quality mental health care into primary care services in resource-limited settings by task shifting skills and responsibilities to community health workers, nurses, physicians, social workers, and psychologists. The ZL team works side by side with a U.S.-trained psychiatrist, the Dr Mario Pagenel Fellow in Global Mental

Table 1
Bio-psycho-social risk and protective factors impacting child mental health in Haiti

	Risk Factors	Protective Factors
Biological	• Lack of prenatal care • Birth trauma and complications • High infant/maternal mortality • Infections • Neurocognitive problems • Physical disabilities • Head trauma • Malnourishment	• Many biological risk factors are preventable and treatable • Mortalities have declined in recent years
Psychological	• Separation from family and corresponding risk of abuse/ neglect • Limited opportunities (education, career) and associated feelings of hopelessness • Sense of danger/mistrust related to prevalence of violence • Poor access to quality education hinders cognitive, emotional, and social development	• Support from extended families and communities • Emphasis on autonomy and liberty • Proud, inspirational history • Cultural/spiritual beliefs (*Voudou*, religion, *lakou*/*konbit* system) that foster strength
Social		
Family/community	• Stigma related to mental and physical illness/disability • Fractured, separated families • Single-parent households • Lack of effective public school system • Lack of safe spaces for children • Parents rendered unable to care for their children	• Extended families and communities provide safety net • Community cohesion tied to religion and spirituality • Emphasis on shared responsibility and concern for peers • Families deeply committed to caring for their children
Poverty and structural violence	• Weakened public sector • Limited economic development and employment opportunities • Lack of effective transportation • Food/water insecurity, malnutrition • Foreign aid apparatus • Vast inequalities in wealth and power • Violence, political instability • Vulnerability to natural disaster	• Aid apparatus can be leveraged to support Haiti's government/ infrastructure • Children represent a powerful, untapped resource for jobs and development • Government's recent efforts to improve child protection
(Mental) health care system	• Limited health care infrastructure • Few resources for children with neurocognitive challenges • Human resources shortage • Services centralized in Port-au-Prince • National health care budget is very limited	• Increased interest in mental health since the earthquake • Greater commitment from MSPP to support mental health and health equity • Promising efforts to develop a sustainable, community-based mental health care system

Box 3
Developing interventions to support and sustain child mental health in Haiti: guiding principles

- Haitian children and their families suffer daily assaults to their well-being but still maintain the strong sense of agency, determination, and hope, which have characterized Haiti since its inception.
- Clinical interventions must build on existing strengths, especially family and community, and interface with community structures, such as church and school, as well as community leaders, including traditional healers.
- Community-based approaches are key to helping patients traverse insurmountable social factors that prevent access to care and keeping children embedded within their families and communities, which often represent the best form of child protection.
- Sustainable models of mental health care must serve all Haitians, especially the 60% who reside in rural regions.
- Haitians themselves must lead efforts, and foreign aid must focus on accompaniment and supporting their leadership, as well as Haiti's public sector, particularly agencies focused on child protection. International actors must consider their actions vis-à-vis Haiti's history of unsuccessful and even damaging foreign interventions.
- Task-shifting, the rational distribution of tasks among health workers, including community health workers, is an effective strategy for addressing Haiti's formidable human resources shortages.
- Developing interventions to support and sustain child mental health in Haiti must address Haiti's larger sociopolitical sphere, which shapes the biological, psychological, and social dimensions shaping children's development and well-being.

Examples of promising interventions/strategies:

- *Zanmi Lasante*: Expansion of a new implementation model to address severe mental disorders in rural Haiti, to inform the development of a national decentralized mental health plan following the 2010 Haiti earthquake
- *Zanmi Lasante*: Teacher-*Accompagnateur* Pilot Study: Pilot test of assessments and implementation and evaluation of a pilot intervention for mental health screening and mental health care access promotion in Haitian schools
- Mercy Corps Moving Forward and Soccer for Life programs

Health Service Delivery, who supports the team through quality improvement efforts and clinical supervision. ZL is working closely with MSPP and has long-term plans to scale-up the model throughout Haiti.[2]

A second successful ZL effort, a mental health *accompagnateur* training for Haitian teachers in secondary schools, has also been developed, implemented, and evaluated. Preliminary findings have indicated that teachers are receptive to developing knowledge and skills related to identifying, responding to, and referring students with mental disorders to services. Moreover, study training was effective in increasing their basic knowledge about and improving attitudes toward mental disorders. School-based mental health screening for major depressive disorder, PTSD, and suicidality was feasible and revealed a high burden of mental disorder or symptoms warranting clinical monitoring. A substantial number of students reported a history of problems accessing health care, and data suggest that many students with mental disorders had not previously accessed care for this problem. Following the earthquake, Mercy Corps, a global aid agency engaged in transitional environments that have experienced some sort of shock, started Moving Forward, a soccer program that uses sports to give vulnerable children a structured environment in which to work through trauma and develop life skills. More than 3100 boys and girls in some of Port-au-Prince's most impoverished neighborhoods have learned how to prevent the spread of HIV/AIDS through the related Soccer for Life program.[76,77] These efforts have demonstrated the feasibility of developing community-based efforts that take advantage of existing structures, like schools, while simultaneously building capacity on other levels, including MSPP. However, few interventions have demonstrated improved clinical or other outcomes, and more research is needed to determine which approaches are most suited to the Haitian context.

ACKNOWLEDGMENTS

The authors wish to thank Eddy Eustache and Giuseppe Raviola for their support in preparing this manuscript.

REFERENCES

1. International Crisis Group. Haiti: stabilisation and reconstruction after the quake. 2010. Available at: http://www.crisisgroup.org/~/media/Files/latin-america/haiti/32_haiti___stabilisation_and_reconstruction_after_the_quake.pdf. Accessed September 26, 2014.
2. Raviola G, Severe J, Therosme T, et al. The 2010 Haiti earthquake response. Psychiatr Clin North Am 2013;36(3):431–50.
3. Kolbe AR, Hutson RA. Human rights abuse and other criminal violations in Port-au-Prince, Haiti: a random survey of households. Lancet 2006;368(9538):864–73.
4. Central Intelligence Agency. The CIA World Factbook Haiti. Updated June 22, 2014. Available at: https://www.cia.gov/library/publications/the-world-factbook/geos/ha.html. Accessed September 26, 2014.
5. Farmer P. The uses of Haiti. Monroe (ME): Common Courage Press; 1994.
6. Dubois L. Haiti: the aftershocks of history. New York: Metropolitan Books;; 2012.
7. Hallward P. Damming the flood: Haiti, Aristide, and the politics of containment. London; New York: Verso; 2007.
8. Malik K. Human development report 2013: the rise of the South: Human progress in a diverse world. Available at: http://hdr.undp.org/en/2013-report.
9. Pierre A, Minn P, Sterlin C, et al. Culture and mental health in Haiti: a literature review. Available at: http://www.who.int/mental_health/emergencies/culture_mental_health_haiti_eng.pdf. Accessed September 26, 2014.
10. Loescher GDSJ. Human rights, U.S. foreign policy, and Haitian refugees. J Inter Am Stud World Aff 1984;26(3):313–56.
11. Doyle M. U.S. Urged to stop Haiti rice subsidies. 2010. Available at: http://www.bbc.co.uk/news/world-latin-america-11472874. Accessed September 26, 2014.
12. Lunde H. Haitian youth survey 2009, volume II: analytical report. Norway: Fafo; 2010.
13. Lunde H. Haiti youth survey 2009, volume I: tablulation report. Norway: Fafo; 2009.
14. Friedman JM, Hagander L, Hughes CD, et al. Distance to hospital and utilization of surgical services in Haiti: do children, delivering mothers, and patients with emergent surgical conditions experience greater geographical barriers to surgical care? Int J Health Plann Manage 2013;28(3):248–56.
15. Lunde H. Youth and education in Haiti disincentives, vulnerabilities and constraints. Published 2008. Avialable at: http://www.fafo.no/pub/rapp/10070/10070.pdf. Accessed September 26, 2014.

16. Schwartz TT. Travesty in Haiti: a true account of Christian missions, orphanages, fraud, food aid and drug trafficking. Charleston (SC): Book Surge Publishing; 2008.
17. Ogzden C, Schiff M. International migration, remittances, and the brain drain. Washington, DC: Palgrave Macmillan; 2006.
18. James EC. Haiti, insecurity, and the politics of asylum. Med Anthropol Q 2011; 25(3):357–76.
19. James EC. The political economy of 'trauma' in Haiti in the democratic era of insecurity. Cult Med Psychiatry 2004;28(2):127–49 [discussion: 211–20].
20. United Nations. Global study on homicide 2013 trends, contexts, data. 2013. Available at: http://www.unodc.org/documents/gsh/pdfs/2014_GLOBAL_HOMICIDE_BOOK_web.pdf. Accessed September 26, 2014.
21. Balsari S, Lemery J, Williams TP, et al. Protecting the children of Haiti. N Engl J Med 2010;362(9):e25.
22. Brennan E. Trying to close orphanages where many aren't orphans at all. New York Times; 2012.
23. Francis J, Reed A, Yohannes F, et al. Screening for tuberculosis among orphans in a developing country. Am J Prev Med 2002;22(2):117–9.
24. Restavek Freedom Website. Available at: restavekfreedom.org. Accessed September 26, 2014.
25. Maurice Sixto. Port-au-Prince (Haiti): Ayitikomik Studios; 2010.
26. Leeds IL, Engel PM, Derby KS, et al. Two cases of restavek-related illness: clinical implications of foster neglect in Haiti. Am J Trop Med Hyg 2010;83(5):1098–9.
27. Suárez LM. The restavèk condition: Jean-Robert Cadet's disclosure. J Haitian Stud 2005;11(1):27–43.
28. Kristof N. A girl's escape. New York Times; 2014.
29. Restavek Freedom. Restavek: the persistence of child labor and slavery. 2011. Available at: http://www.ijdh.org/wp-content/uploads/2011/03/Haiti-UPR-Restavek-Report-FINAL1.pdf. Accessed September 26, 2014.
30. Nicolas G, Schwartz B, Pierre E. Weathering the storms like bamboo: the strengths of Haitians in coping with natural disasters. In: Kalayjian AED, editor. Mass trauma and emotional healing around the world rituals and practices for resilience and meaning-making. Santa Barbara (CA): Praeger; 2010. p. 93–106.
31. N'Zengou-Tayo M. 'Fanm se poto mitan': Haitian woman, the pillar of society. Fem Rev 1998;(59):118–42.
32. Alexandre PK, Saint-Jean G, Crandall L, et al. Prenatal care utilization in rural areas and urban areas of Haiti. Rev Panam Salud Publica 2005;18(2):84–92.
33. Lomotey CJ, Lewis J, Gebrian B, et al. Maternal and congenital syphilis in rural Haiti. Rev Panam Salud Publica 2009;26(3):197–202.
34. Fitzgerald DW, Behets FM, Lucet C, et al. Prevalence, burden, and control of syphilis in Haiti's rural Artibonite region. Int J Infect Dis 1998;2(3):127–31.
35. Hossain SK, Porter EL, Redden LM, et al. Maternity waiting home use and maternal mortality in Milot, Haiti. Obstet Gynecol 2014;123(Suppl 1):149S.
36. Small MJ, Gupta J, Frederic R, et al. Intimate partner and nonpartner violence against pregnant women in rural Haiti. Int J Gynaecol Obstet 2008;102(3): 226–31.
37. Pan American Health Organization. Haiti: profile of the health services system. 2003. Available at: http://new.paho.org/hq/dmdocuments/2010/Health_System_Profile-Haiti_2003.pdf. Accessed September 26, 2014.
38. Koenig S, Ivers L, Pace S, et al. Successes and challenges of HIV treatment programs in Haiti: aftermath of the earthquake. HIV Ther 2010;4(2):145–60.

39. Ayoya MA, Heidkamp R, Ngnie-Teta I, et al. Précis of nutrition of children and women in Haiti: analyses of data from 1995 to 2012. Ann N Y Acad Sci 2014; 1309:37–62.
40. Heidkamp RA, Ngnie-Teta I, Ayoya MA, et al. Predictors of anemia among Haitian children aged 6 to 59 months and women of childbearing age and their implications for programming. Food Nutr Bull 2013;34(4):462–79.
41. Martsolf DS. Childhood maltreatment and mental and physical health in Haitian adults. J Nurs Scholarsh 2004;36(4):293–9.
42. Douyon R, Herns Marcelin L, Jean-Gilles M, et al. Response to trauma in Haitian youth at risk. J Ethn Subst Abuse 2005;4(2):115–38.
43. Fawzi MC, Betancourt TS, Marcelin L, et al. Depression and post-traumatic stress disorder among Haitian immigrant students: implications for access to mental health services and educational programming. BMC Public Health 2009;9:482.
44. Lunde H. The violent lifeworlds of young Haitians: Gangs as livelihood in a Port-au-Prince ghetto. Norway: Fafo; 2012.
45. Lunde H. Young Haitian labour migrants risks and opportunities in Haiti and the Dominican Republic. Norway: Fafo; 2010.
46. Gupta J, Agrawal A. Chronic aftershocks of an earthquake on the well-being of children in Haiti: violence, psychosocial health and slavery. Can Med Assoc J 2010;182(18):1997–9.
47. Smith Fawzi MC, Eustache E, Oswald C, et al. Psychosocial functioning among HIV-affected youth and their caregivers in Haiti: implications for family-focused service provision in high HIV burden settings. Aids Patient Care STDS 2010; 24(3):147–58.
48. Surkan PJ, Mukherjee JS, Williams DR, et al. Perceived discrimination and stigma toward children affected by HIV/AIDS and their HIV-positive caregivers in central Haiti. AIDS Care 2010;22(7):803–15.
49. Gomez AM, Speizer IS, Beauvais H. Sexual violence and reproductive health among youth in Port-au-Prince, Haiti. J Adolesc Health 2009;44(5):508–10.
50. Wagenaar BH, Hagaman AK, Kaiser BN, et al. Depression, suicidal ideation, and associated factors: a cross-sectional study in rural Haiti. BMC Psychiatry 2012; 12:149.
51. Birbeck GL. Epilepsy care in developing countries: part I of II. Epilepsy Curr 2010;10(4):75–9.
52. World Health Organization. Le Systeme de Sante Mental en Haiti. Available at: http://www.who.int/mental_health/who_aims_country_reports/who_aims_report_haiti_fr.pdf. Accessed September 26. 2014.
53. Sontag D. Haiti, mental health system is in collapse. New York Times; 2010.
54. Nicolas G, Jean-Jacques R, Wheatley A. Mental health counseling in Haiti: historical overview, current status, and plans for the future. J Black Psychol 2012;38(4): 509–19.
55. Schwartz B, Bernal D, Smith L, et al. Pathways to understand help-seeking behaviors among Haitians. J Immigr Minor Health 2014;16(2):239–43.
56. Carrazana E, DeToledo J, Tatum W, et al. Epilepsy and religious experiences: voodoo possession. Epilepsia 1999;40(2):239–41.
57. Cavanna AE, Cavanna S, Cavanna A. Epileptic seizures and spirit possession in Haitian culture: report of four cases and review of the literature. Epilepsy Behav 2010;19(1):89–91.
58. Wagenaar BH, Kohrt BA, Hagaman AK, et al. Determinants of care seeking for mental health problems in rural Haiti: culture, cost, or competency. Psychiatr Serv 2013;64(4):366–72.

59. Kobetz E, Menard J, Kish J, et al. Impacts of the 2010 Haitian earthquake in the diaspora: findings from Little Haiti, Miami, FL. J Immigr Minor Health 2013;15(2):442–7.
60. Nicolas G, Desilva AM, Subrebost KL, et al. Expression and treatment of depression among Haitian immigrant women in the United States: clinical observations. Am J Psychother 2007;61(1):83–98.
61. Keys HM, Kaiser BN, Kohrt BA, et al. Idioms of distress, ethnopsychology, and the clinical encounter in Haiti's Central Plateau. Soc Sci Med 2012;75(3):555–64.
62. Khoury NM, Kaiser BN, Keys HM, et al. Explanatory models and mental health treatment: is vodou an obstacle to psychiatric treatment in rural Haiti? Cult Med Psychiatry 2012;36(3):514–34.
63. Disasters Emergency Committee. Haiti earthquake facts and figures. Available at: http://www.dec.org.uk/haiti-earthquake-facts-and-figures. Accessed September 26, 2014.
64. IASC. Response to the Humanitarian Crisis in Haiti Following the 12 January 2010 earthquake: achievements, challenges, and lessons to be learned. Available at: https://www.ifrc.org/docs/IDRL/Haiti/IASC-Haiti_6Mos_Review_USA-2010-005-1.pdf. Accessed September 26. 2014.
65. Bar-On E, Lebel E, Blumberg N, et al. Pediatric orthopedic injuries following an earthquake: experience in an acute-phase field hospital. J Trauma Acute Care Surg 2013;74(2):617–21.
66. Farfel A, Assa A, Amir I, et al. Haiti earthquake 2010: a field hospital pediatric perspective. Eur J Pediatr 2011;170(4):519–25.
67. Kelley M. Should international adoption be part of humanitarian aid efforts? Lessons from Haiti. Bioethics 2010;24(7):373–80.
68. Institute for Justice and Democracy in Haiti. Gender-based violence against Haitian women and girls in internal displacement camps, submission to the United Nations. Available at: http://ijdh.org/wordpress/wp-content/uploads/2011/03/UPR-GBV-Final-4-4-2011.pdf. Accessed September 26. 2014.
69. Center for Human Rights and Global Justice. Sexual violence in Haiti's IDP camps: results of a household survey. Available at: http://chrgj.org/wp-content/uploads/2012/07/HaitiSexualViolenceMarch2011.pdf. Accessed September 26. 2014.
70. UNICEF. UNICEF Annual report for Haiti 2010. Available at: http://www.unicef.org/about/annualreport/files/Haiti_COAR_2010.pdf. Accessed September 26, 2014.
71. Ghosh B. Haiti's mass graveyard of old and new nightmares. Time; 2010.
72. Cenat JM, Derivois D. Assessment of prevalence and determinants of posttraumatic stress disorder and depression symptoms in adults survivors of earthquake in Haiti after 30 months. J Affect Disord 2014;159:111–7.
73. Inter Agency Standing Committee. Guidance note for mental health and psychosocial support. 2010. Available at: https://www.k4health.org/sites/default/files/haiti_guidance_note_mhpss.pdf.
74. United Nations. Haiti: six months after. Available at: http://www.un.org/en/peacekeeping/missions/minustah/documents/6_months_after_commemoration.pdf. Accessed September 26. 2014.
75. Sontag D. Rebuilding in Haiti lags after billions in post-quake aid. New York Times; 2012.
76. Save the Children. Haiti four years after: towards a lasting legacy for Haitian children. Available at: http://ijdh.org/wordpress/wp-content/uploads/2011/03/UPR-GBV-Final-4-4-2011.pdf. Accessed September 26, 2014.
77. Mercy Corps. Giving kids a sporting chance. Available at: http://www.mercycorps.org/articles/haiti/giving-kids-sporting-chance. Accessed September 26, 2014.

Implicit Cognition

Implications for Global Health Disparities

Neha A. John-Henderson, PhD

KEYWORDS

- Implicit cognition • Implicit bias • Social inequalities in health
- Patient-physician relationship • Global health

KEY POINTS

- Implicit measures of cognition are not equivalent to our explicitly endorsed beliefs.
- Implicit beliefs and biases predict measures of physical and mental health independently of explicit beliefs.
- Implicit biases interact with demographic variables and daily experiences to predict markers of health.
- Implicit biases held by both patient and physician influence communication, perceptions of quality of care, and treatment decisions.

As humans, we are inclined to believe that our conscious thoughts and beliefs shape our behavior and decisions. However, implicit cognition, or our unconscious attitudes, beliefs, and biases, is also a powerful shaper of our actions. These implicit beliefs or associations are activated without intention or awareness, and everyone possesses them regardless of their socioeconomic status (SES), gender, race, or age.[1] Our early life experiences begin the shaping of these implicit cognitions, and they continue to develop over the course of the lifespan informed directly and indirectly through our experiences, the media, and observing the behavior of others.[2,3] Although these implicit cognitions have wide-reaching effects, this article focuses on ways in which they can affect mental and physical health, contribute to health disparities, and affect the patient-physician relationship and treatment decisions.

IMPLICIT VERSUS EXPLICIT

Before discussing specific ways in which implicit cognitions can affect health, it is important to understand the difference between implicit and explicit measures of

---

Disclosures: The author declared no potential conflicts of interest with respect to the authorship and/or publication of this article.
Department of Psychology, University of Pittsburgh, 4405 Sennott Square, 201 South Bouquet Street, Pittsburgh, PA 15213, USA
E-mail address: neha.jh@pitt.edu

Child Adolesc Psychiatric Clin N Am 24 (2015) 751–763
http://dx.doi.org/10.1016/j.chc.2015.06.005 **childpsych.theclinics.com**
1056-4993/15/$ – see front matter

cognition. Explicit cognitions are typically associated with deliberate responses that are within an individual's control, whereas implicit measures capture attitudes, beliefs, or personal and cultural biases that exist outside of our conscious awareness. Given this distinction, our implicit associations do not necessarily align with the beliefs or associations that we explicitly endorse.[4] However, they are not mutually exclusive and may in fact work to reinforce one another. Both are significant, and neither should be considered the sole authentic measure of cognition.[5]

IMPLICIT MEASURES OF BIAS

> *Implicit biases come from the culture. I think of them as the thumbprint of the culture on our minds. Human beings have the ability to learn to associate two things together very quickly—that is innate. What we teach ourselves, what we choose to associate is up to us.*
>
> —*Dr Mahzarin Banaji.*

An implicit bias is a discriminatory bias that is largely based on implicit attitudes or stereotypes and can be either favorable or unfavorable. With regards to biases about social groups, in-group bias designates favoritism toward ones' own social group, whereas out-group bias is a negative bias toward individuals from another social group.[6] Implicit measures of bias are particularly important and informative with respect to topics that are politically, culturally, or socially sensitive (eg, race, gender, religion, obesity). For example, accurately capturing racial attitudes of Americans presents a significant challenge as respondents are motivated to answer in such a way that indicates the absence of racial bias.[6] As such, implicit measures of bias may offer a more accurate examination of the relationship between our beliefs and biases in these domains and health outcomes.

As a result of repeated reinforcement of social stereotypes, these implicit biases take root early in life.[7] Evidence suggests that explicit beliefs about race become more egalitarian with age, whereas implicit beliefs remain unchanged,[8] and it is possible that implicit and explicit beliefs about other demographic variables or traits may follow similar trajectories. These implicit biases are powerful shapers of our daily behaviors and actions. For example, in a sample of college students, implicit racial bias had no relation to self-reported egalitarian values; however, they predicted perceived friendliness in interactions with a black student.[9]

CAPTURING THE IMPLICIT

Because these implicit measures cannot be captured with traditional self-report, social psychologists, borrowing methods from cognitive psychology, developed the Implicit Association Test (IAT). The IAT assesses the ease or difficulty with which the mind makes associations. Based on the understanding that learning is a result of changes in neural function of different neurons that are active at the same time, the cognitive principle that the IAT is based on is that concepts in the mind that are closely associated with each other are more closely linked.[10] These associations can occur for unconscious processes in addition to conscious processes. Although there are other instruments used to obtain implicit measures, this discussion focuses on the IAT because it is the task most commonly used for this purpose.

More specifically, the IAT measures relative strengths of automatic associations between 2 contrasted target concepts and 2 attribute concepts. Words from all 4 concept categories appear in the middle of a computer screen in mixed order. Individuals taking the IAT are instructed to sort the words with a left (Q) or right (P) response key.[10,11] The idea is that the sorting task is easier when a target and an attribute are strongly associated than when they are weakly associated. For example, a clinically depressed person should find it easier to categorize words in the category of me and words in the category of depressed than they would for words in the category of me with words in the category of happy. The category labels are visible throughout the duration of the task in the upper left and right corners of the screen. Several examples of the IAT task are available on the Project Implicit Web site: https://implicit.harvard.edu/implicit.

Evidence for the unique contribution of implicit measures comes from a meta-analysis of the predictive validity of the IAT. The analyses of 122 research studies that used the IAT provided evidence that, although explicit and implicit measures have unique predictive validity for behavioral, judgment, and physiologic measures, the predictive validity of explicit measures for these outcomes is significantly impaired for socially sensitive topics, highlighting an important contribution of implicit measures.[10]

Research using the IAT demonstrates that these unconscious associations and beliefs can be formed about many phenomena, including the self, memories, others, and inanimate objects. For example, if one was interested in measuring implicit attitudes, the self as being sad or happy, the concepts would be *sad* words (eg, miserable, depressed), *happy* words (eg, joyful, content), *me* words (eg, my, I), and *other* words (eg, them, they).[12] **Fig. 1** displays a visual representation of 2 screens from the IAT described earlier.

IMPLICIT MEASURES AND MENTAL HEALTH

During the last 2 decades, there has been a growing interest in implicit associations and their impact on psychopathology.[13] Explicit cognitions are strongly predictive of controlled behaviors, whereas automatic associations are more closely associated with spontaneous uncontrollable behaviors.[14] The latter of these behaviors are involved in psychopathology whereby patients often report symptoms being unpredictable and out of their control. Changes in explicit associations induced by treatment are independent of changes in automatic associations.[15] As such, automatic associations that are not affected by treatment could in part explain the persistence of psychopathologic symptoms.

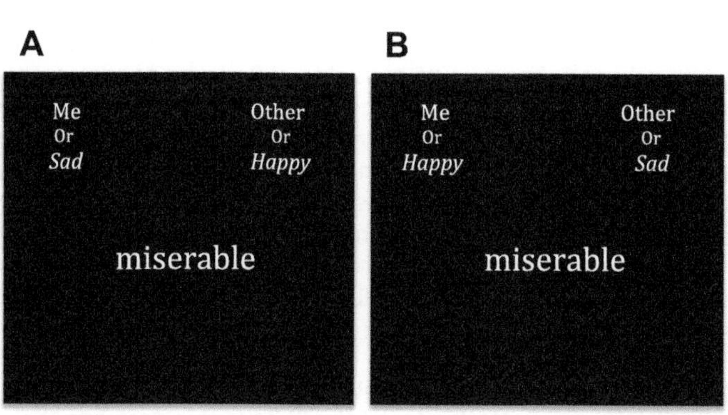

Fig. 1. Visual representation of an IAT testing associations between the self and happy or sad. (*A*) EASIER. (*B*) HARDER. Panels (*A*) and (*B*) are examples of the contrasts of associations that would be easier versus harder to make for an individual who more strongly associated themselves with being sad than being happy.

Several studies provide evidence of a relationship between automatic self-associations and various types of psychopathologic symptoms. For example, automatic self-anxious associations are involved in anxiety and anxious behavior.[16] Research has shown that beyond these relationships, different self-associations are uniquely predictive of distinct disorders independently of parallel explicit measures of self-associations. In a study of 2329 Dutch patients, individuals with anxiety disorder showed stronger automatic self-anxious associations than did depressed patients and controls, whereas depressed patients showed stronger automatic self-depressed associations than anxious patients and controls. Furthermore, these automatic associations significantly predicted the severity of anxious and depressive symptoms more than explicit self-beliefs.[17]

Treatment-Induced Changes in Automatic Associations

Given these associations between automatic associations and psychopathologic symptoms, the question arises as to whether these automatic associations are affected by treatment and whether these changes correspond with reduction in severity of symptoms. One study explored this question in the context of panic disorder. Individuals with panic disorder underwent 12 weeks of cognitive behavior therapy (CBT) and completed an IAT measuring implicit associations between the concepts panicked and calm and me and not me once every 3 weeks over the course of the CBT. Their findings suggest that changes in implicit associations between the self and panic not only change over the course of CBT for panic disorder but also predict change in panic symptom severity.[18] This study provides insight into an important mechanism by which CBT can affect the trajectory of symptom severity in the context of panic disorder. An important extension of this work is an examination of how treatment of other disorders affects implicit self-associations and the degree to which these changes are predictive of the trajectory of symptom severity for affected individuals.

Implicit Associations and Suicide Ideation

Suicide is the third leading cause of death among adolescents in the United States, and the causes of suicidal behaviors are not fully understood with the rates of death by suicide remaining flat.[19] Furthermore, suicide is difficult to predict because clinical assessment relies on the individual choosing to self-report suicidal thoughts, and individuals with these thoughts are often motivated to conceal them. One study tested whether implicit associations between self-injury and oneself predicted suicide ideation and suicide attempts. The sample consisted of 3 groups of adolescents: nonsuicidal individuals, suicide ideators, and recent suicide attempters. There were large between-group differences on the self-injury IAT with suicide ideators showing small positive associations between self-injury and the self and suicide attempters showing large positive associations on this test. This test accurately predicted current suicide ideation and attempt status as well as future suicide ideation. In addition, it improved prediction of these outcomes more than known risk factors.[20] Thus, measures of these implicit associations could be an invaluable tool in the effort to prevent suicidal behavior and deaths.

IMPLICIT BIASES AND PHYSICAL HEALTH OUTCOMES

Implicit Social Class Bias as a Moderator of the Relationship Between Socioeconomic Status and Health

SES is one of the most robust predictors of health and well-being globally.[21] Consistently, for numerous diseases and mental and physical health outcomes, an inverse relationship between SES and health has been documented. This relationship is not observed only at the extremes of the SES distributions. Instead, each increment in SES is associated with better health. Traditionally, objective indicators such as years of education, occupation, and income have been used to measure an individual's SES. More recently, attention has been given to the importance of subjective perceptions of SES.[21] The MacArthur scale of subjective social status is a commonly used measure to assess subjective perceptions of SES. In this measure, individuals are asked to place an X indicating where they place themselves on a 10-rung ladder relative to others in the United States (**Fig. 2**). This subjective measure of SES has been shown to be predictive of mental and physical health outcomes, independent of traditional markers of SES.[21,22]

Despite this strong relationship, some individuals from low SES backgrounds demonstrate resilience and exhibit profiles of health similar to their high SES counterparts, which is of particular importance because large numbers of the populations in many parts of the world are by and large impoverished and poor and yet resilient. One investigation examined the extent to which a person's implicit attitude about social

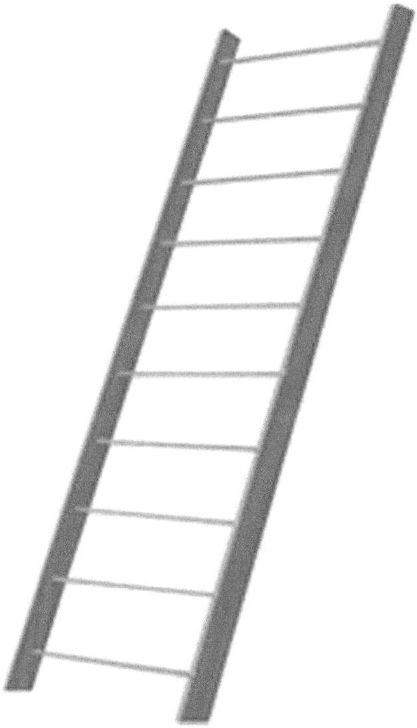

Fig. 2. The MacArthur scale of subjective social status. Participants are shown the ladder and respond to the following prompt: Think of this ladder as representing where people stand in the United States. At the top of the ladder are the people who are the best off, those who have the most money, the most education, and the most respected jobs. At the bottom are the people who are the worst off, who have the least money, the least education, and the least respected jobs or no job. The higher up you are on this ladder, the closer you are to the people at the very top; the lower you are, the closer you are to the people at the very bottom. Where would you place yourself on this ladder? Please place a large X on the rung where you think you stand at this time in your life, relative to other people in the United States.

class (automatic evaluative associations about social class) coupled with their subjective perception of their social status affected a marker of inflammation within the immune system. The findings revealed that individuals who thought that they were low on the ladder relative to others in the United States (ie, low subjective social status) who also harbored high levels of implicit social class bias (ie, strong associations between lower class and bad) exhibited the greatest levels of the proinflammatory cytokine interleukin (IL) 6 (**Fig. 3**).[22] Elevated levels of IL-6 are implicated in numerous disease processes,[23] and the differences observed in a young, healthy sample, could indicate different health trajectories emerging as a function of these psychosocial factors. In this research, explicit social class bias was related to current depressive symptoms and self-rated health, whereas only implicit social class bias predicted levels of circulating IL-6.[22]

Racial Disparities in Health and the Role of Implicit Biases

African American men experience disproportionately greater rates of chronic disease and accelerated declines in health compared with other racial and gender groups in the United States.[24] These racial disparities in health may be in part a result of a greater number of psychosocial stressors, particularly those tied to their racial minority status.[25] A large body of research documents the stressful nature of experiences of

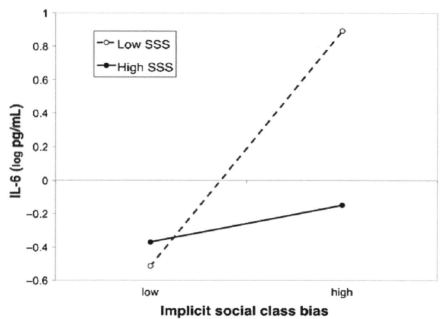

Fig. 3. Implicit social class bias moderated the effect of subjective social status (SSS) on IL-6 levels. There was a significant interaction between implicit social class bias and subjective social status on circulating levels of IL-6 ($P<.001$; 95% confidence interval, −0.417, −0.117). IL-6 values are reported as standardized values of log-transformed IL-6 values (picograms per milliliter). Analyses controlled for objective SES. All variables were measured and analyzed as continuous variables. Plotted values represent predicted scores for participants 1 standard deviation more and less than the implicit social class bias and subjective social class distributions. (*From* John-Henderson N, Jacobs EG, Mendoza-Denton R, et al. Wealth, health and the moderating role of implicit social class bias. Ann Behav Med 2013;45:177; with permission.)

discrimination in daily life.[26] These stressful experiences could affect physical health through mental health pathways or by shaping health behaviors.[27] Negative evaluations of one's own racial group could contribute additional psychosocial stress and thus may moderate the effects of experiences of racial discrimination on health. Here, 2 ways in which implicit racial biases have been shown to predict important markers of physical health are discussed.

One line of research focused on the interactive effects of racial discrimination and implicit racial biases among African American men on an important marker of aging at the biological level. Telomeres are repetitive sequences of DNA located at the end of the body's chromosomes that are important in protecting against DNA degradation and promotion of chromosomal stability. In eukaryotes, with each mitotic cycle, telomere attrition occurs. As such, telomere length is viewed as a marker of aging at the cellular level.[28] Leukocyte telomere length (LTL) is associated with several aging-related disorders and diseases such as cardiovascular disease and dementia.[29,30] Psychosocial stressors have been related to accelerated LTL shortening,[31] suggesting a potential mechanism by which experiences and biases related to racial identity could contribute to racial disparities in health. In line with this, in a sample of African American men, after controlling for actual age and socioeconomic and health-related characteristics, those individuals who reported higher levels of racial discrimination and exhibited internalization of in-group racial bias (ie, implicit association between African American and bad) exhibited the shortest LTL.[32]

A parallel line of research focused on how these processes contribute to racial disparities in cardiovascular health between African American and white men that are well documented.[33] Research examining the role of experiences of racial discrimination as a predictor of hypertension risk has been largely inconsistent. Some studies have found no association between self-reports of racial discrimination and cardiovascular health, whereas others have found moderated or curvilinear relationships. Increasing evidence suggests that social stressors and psychosocial challenges play a critical role in heightening vulnerability to cardiovascular disease for African American men.[34] One investigation explored the role of implicit racial bias in this relationship. The findings suggested that among African American men, the combination of experiencing racial discrimination and holding an implicit antiblack bias was associated with a higher probability of hypertension, whereas among those with an implicit pro-black bias, it was associated with lower risk.[35]

Implications for Obesity

The discrimination and stigmatization associated with obesity is pervasive and is stronger today than it was 40 years ago.[36] Overweight and obese individuals face significant social disadvantages in almost every domain of life.[37] Somewhat ironically, the social distress associated with this disadvantage is believed to worsen or even cause adiposity-related disorders and as a result could heighten both perceived and actual experiences of discrimination and stigmatization.[38] In contrast to more historically acknowledged dimensions of identity that are associated with stigmatization (eg, race and gender), there are no legal sanctions in place to protect individuals from what is now referred to as obese-ism.[39]

Antifat bias refers to the prejudicial assumption that a person who appears to be obese must also have negative personality traits (eg, lazy, greedy, unmotivated). Using an IAT, one study demonstrated that strong implicit antifat attitudes exist despite the lack of an explicit antifat bias.[40] In an online sample of 4283 individuals, implicit antifat bias was moderately strong even among extremely obese individuals. However, the researchers noted that the magnitude of the antifat bias was smaller for more obese individuals.[40] In addition, this research highlighted the somewhat alarming fact that a substantial portion of the sample was willing to endure aversive life events to avoid being obese. These studies are examples from a growing literature that highlight the pervasiveness of antifat biases at an implicit level. This work should be extended in 2 important ways. First, given that social distress can contribute and exacerbate adiposity-related disease, it is possible that the degree of implicit antifat bias that an obese individual holds could predict change in body mass over time and overall health. In addition, future work should examine whether the degree of implicit antifat biases affects the behaviors, coping, and lifestyle choices of obese individuals. For example, does a stronger antifat implicit bias promote healthy dietary choices and more frequent exercise, or would it discourage obese individuals from making changes that could improve their physical and mental health?

IMPLICIT BIASES IN A HEALTH CARE SETTING

The ways in which these implicit cognitions can affect health at the level of the individual were discussed. A parallel line of research provides substantial evidence that implicit biases among health care professionals exist and can contribute to already existing health disparities.[41,42] These implicit biases can shape physician behavior in a way that produces differential medical treatment as a function of race, gender, ethnicity, or other individual characteristics.

The IAT has been used to measure the degree to which these implicit biases exist among physicians. Using data from Harvard's Project Implicit Web site, one study showed individuals with an MD degree exhibit an implicit preference for thin people and that this bias was similar to the level observed among the general public.[43] Similarly, another investigation revealed in a sample of 2535 medical doctors a strong implicit bias in favor of white Americans relative to black Americans.[44]

How do these biases in turn affect patient-doctor interactions? As a first pathway, evidence suggests that implicit biases may shape patient-doctor communication. One investigation specifically explored how physicians' implicit racial biases affect communication and care and how these biases predicted patients' perception of care. In this study, white and Asian physicians overall held more prowhite attitudes than did African American physicians. After coding patient-physician interactions, the investigators reported that physician racial bias (ie, favoring whites) was associated with greater clinician domination of the dialogue for patients of all races and a less positive patient emotional tone in visits with African Americans. Physician racial bias predicted patients' reports of their experience with their physician. African American patients who were seen by physicians who exhibited stronger implicit preference for whites reported less confidence in their clinicians care, perceived less respect from their physician, liked their doctors less, and reported that they were less likely to recommend their doctor to a friend.[45]

This study also investigated whether physicians hold implicit racial stereotypes about whether a patient's race affects the likelihood that they will comply with medical advice. Physicians who held the implicit stereotype that African American patients are less compliant with medical advice spent more time with African American patients than with white patients. These longer visits were characterized by slower speech speed; physician-dominated interactions; less attention to the social, psychological, and emotional issues related to the patients' condition and care; and lower levels of positive tone compared with their visits with white patients.[45] Although one could argue that these longer visits could be a sign of an increased effort to connect with the patient, African American patients' response to these visits was negative.

Together, these findings provide compelling evidence that implicit biases affect the bidirectional relationship between patient and physician and could affect the patients' confidence and trust in their physician and their compliance to medical advice.

An important question arises from these findings: Do these implicit biases also affect treatment decisions and thus directly affect patient health? One line of research provides evidence that treatment decisions are influenced by patient ethnicity or race. In one study, Hispanic patients were 7 times less likely to receive opioids in the emergency room than non-Hispanic patients with similar injuries,[46] and these findings were duplicated for black patients.[47] As an extension of this work, another investigation examined whether there were differences in physicians' ability to accurately judge the severity of patient pain as a function of race. The findings revealed that, although there were no differences in accuracy of pain perception as a function of patient ethnicity, Hispanic patients with severe injuries were still given less analgesia.[48] These investigations do not directly measure implicit bias but find that physicians make differential treatment decisions for patients with similar clinical presentations who differ in ethnicity or race.

A separate line of research directly measures physicians' implicit biases and examines the relationship between these biases and treatment decisions. In one study, medical residents took the black/white, good/bad IAT and answered questions about a vignette describing a patient that was randomly designated as being black or white. Residents who exhibited greater implicit prowhite bias were significantly less likely to recommend thrombolysis for the treatment of acute coronary syndromes for black patients than those with less bias.[49] Although this study revealed differential treatment of hypothetical patients, the pattern reflects a real-life health care disparity in that black patients with acute coronary syndrome are less likely to receive appropriate therapies than white patients with acute coronary syndrome.[50]

A review on the current understanding of implicit bias and health disparities in health care settings notes that health disparities exist among multiple social dimensions and so future investigations should give attention to the degree to which implicit biases exist for each of these groups.[51] Furthermore, patients are not members of only one social group. Instead, they simultaneously belong to a race/ethnic group, a sex group, and an age group. Whether and how implicit biases for or against these groups interact is unexplored. At the same time, less is known about how implicit biases held by the patient could affect their relationship with the clinician and consequently shape compliance and communication. Implicit biases existing on both ends of the patient-physician relationship could inhibit communication and trust and therefore impede treatment and adversely affect the health of the patient.

DISCUSSION

There is a growing and diverse literature that seeks to unpack the relationship between implicit cognitions and health-related outcomes. As evidenced by research, implicit cognitions are associated with both mental and physical health outcomes and could affect health by shaping the nature of the patient-physician relationships and could even affect treatment decisions.

At the level of the individual, these findings indicate that harboring an implicit in-group negative bias interacts with daily experiences and psychosocial factors to predict important markers of health and vulnerability. Individuals with implicit biases against their own social group may be more inclined to believe they are responsible in part for negative experiences and may be increasingly vulnerable to stigmatizing experiences. This heightened vulnerability may be evident in heightened psychological and physiologic reactivity to stressors, which over time could contribute to allostatic load and increased risk for numerous diseases.[52]

Although the association between these implicit biases and biological markers of risk has been documented cross-sectionally, less is known about the pathways through which implicit biases affect markers of health and disease in daily life. An important future direction for this body of research will be investigations of how these implicit biases manifest in daily life in the form of emotional responses, behavioral responses (eg, substance abuse, food consumption, smoking), and physiologic responses. This research would afford the opportunity to design interventions that could manage or reduce the frequency of problematic responses that could exacerbate risk for ill-health.

At the same time, a summary of studies examining the malleability of implicit biases provides ample evidence that these biases are in fact plastic, thus revealing another promising point of intervention. For example, implicit gender stereotypes of feminine weakness were reduced simply by asking participants to imagine examples of women who challenged this stereotype,[53] and implicit antiblack race bias was reduced by having an African American experimenter administer the IAT.[54] By and large, these studies show that although implicit biases can be reduced, they are generally not eliminated. It is possible that what is occurring in this research is a temporary activation of a subtype of a larger category. As such, these studies cannot speak to the permanence of these changes. Longitudinal research addressing the stability of these reductions in bias will provide important direction when considering how best to affect these biases in a durable and meaningful manner.

Another important consideration in reducing the existence and degree of implicit biases and their consequent effects on health is an understanding of the developmental substantiation of these biases. We know that these biases emerge early in life, and our understanding is that they are a product of exposures in our environment. The images we see on television, the stories we hear, and our observation of social interactions of those close to us, are all important informants of our beliefs and biases. More research is warranted so that we can better understand which influences matter most and when in the development of these unconscious biases.

With regards to implicit biases in the context of health care, the most obvious point of intervention would be an attempt to modify or reduce any unconscious biases or stereotypes held by physicians. The first step in this process would be to provide evidence of these implicit cognitions. However, even if physicians are convinced that they should feel differently and they are motivated to change the bias, it does not guarantee that the bias will be reduced or eliminated. In fact, evidence suggests that directly trying to suppress biases only has a temporary effect on the bias, which reappears at a later time.[55] Promoting awareness of these biases may be effective in directing attention to whether there are differences in behavior and communication with patients as a function of their social group or other defining characteristics and could be a significant contribution to the overarching goal of reducing social disparities in health.

Moving forward, effort should be made to ensure that implicit beliefs, associations, and biases are included in investigations that strive to investigate the role of cognitive processes in predicting health outcomes, both in the general public and in the context of a health care setting. For the latter, measures should be collected for both patient and medical provider, and investigations will need to expand beyond the most commonly studied social groups (African American and female patients) to explore how other populations are affected by these biases. The findings from this line of research should inform policy in all health care settings globally, in a way that supports initiatives to improve recognition of disparities in treatment that may be rooted in unconscious biases. In addition, there is evidence that increasing diversity in the population of health care providers may work to attenuate automatic racial biases, merely by increasing exposure to individuals from social groups that are traditionally underrepresented in these settings.[56]

This line of research has structured investigations in a way that views mental and physical health outcomes as largely distinct. As noted in the Milliman report,[57] physical and mental health are related and optimal financial and clinical outcomes are achieved when care for mental and physical health is coordinated. As such, future investigations should use a more global, comprehensive examination of the ways in which implicit biases affect both mental and physical outcomes of health. In conclusion, as noted by Blair and colleagues,[58] although implicit bias is pervasive, there are certainly some individuals who do not show any implicit bias on specific measures. An exploration of the factors that make these individuals less vulnerable to implicit biases is worthy of investigation and could reduce the overall impact of implicit biases on health, both at the level of the individual and by positively affecting the relationship between patient and physician.

REFERENCES

1. Nosek BA, Smyth FL, Hansen JJ, et al. Pervasiveness and correlates of implicit attitudes and stereotypes. Eur Rev Soc Psychol 2007;18:36–88.
2. Dasgupta N. Implicit attitudes and beliefs adapt to situations: a decade of research on the malleability of implicit prejudice, stereotypes, and the self-concept. Adv Exp Soc Psychol 2013;47:233–79.
3. Rudman LA. Sources of implicit attitudes. Curr Dir Psychol Sci 2004;13:79–82.
4. Graham S, Lowery BS. Priming unconscious stereotypes about adolescent offenders. Law Hum Behav 2004;28:483–504.
5. Krieger N, Carney D, Lancaster K, et al. Combining explicit and implicit measures of racial discrimination in health research. Am J Public Health 2010;100:1485–92.
6. McConahay JB, Hardee BB, Batts V. Has racism declined in America? It depends on who is asking and what is asked? J Conflict Resolut 1981;25:563–79.
7. Dunham Y, Baron AS, Banaji MR. From American city to Japanese village: a cross-cultural investigation of implicit race attitudes. Child Dev 2006;77:1268–81.
8. Baron AS, Banaji MR. The development of implicit attitudes. Evidence of race evaluations from ages 6 and 10 and adulthood. Psychol Sci 2006;17:53–8.
9. Dovidio JF, Kawakami K, Gaertner SL. Implicit and explicit prejudice and interracial interaction. J Pers Soc Psychol 2002;82:62–8.
10. Greenwald AG, Poehlman AT, Uhlmann EL, et al. Understanding and using the Implicit Association Test. III. Meta-analysis of predictive validity. J Pers Soc Psychol 2009;97:17–41.
11. Greenwald AG, Banaji MR. Implicit social cognition: attitudes, self-esteem, and stereotypes. Psychol Rev 1995;102:4–27.
12. Nosek BA, Greenwald AG, Banaji MR. The implicit association test at age 7: a methodological and conceptual review. In: Bargh JA, editor. Automatic processes in social thinking and behavior. New York: Psychology Press; 2007. p. 265–92.
13. De Houwer J. The implicit association test as a tool for studying dysfunctional associations in psychopathology: strengths and limitations. J Behav Ther Exp Psychiatry 2002;33:115–33.
14. Huijding J, de Jong PJ. Specific predictive power of automatic spider-related affective associations for controllable and uncontrollable fear responses towards spiders. Behav Res Ther 2006;44:161–76.

15. Huijding J, de Jong PJ. Implicit and explicit attitudes towards spiders: sensitivity to treatment and predictive validity for generalization of treatment effects. Cognit Ther Res 2009;33:211–20.
16. Egloff B, Schmulke SC. Predictive validity of an implicit association test for assessing anxiety. J Pers Soc Psychol 2002;83:1441–55.
17. Glashouwer K, de Jong PJ. Disorder-specific automatic self-associations in anxiety and depression: results of the Netherlands study of depression and anxiety. Psychol Med 2010;40:1101–11.
18. Teachman BA, Marker CD, Smith-Janik SB. Automatic associations and panic disorder: trajectories of change over the course of treatment. J Consult Clin Psychol 2008;76:988–1002.
19. Centers for Disease Control and Prevention. Youth risk behavior surveillance-United States, 2011. MMWR Surveill Summ 2012;61(4):1–162.
20. Nock MK, Banaji MR. Prediction of suicide ideation and attempts among adolescents using a brief performance-based test. J Consult Clin Psychol 2007;75:707–15.
21. Operario D, Adler NE, Williams DR. Subjective social status: reliability and predictive utility for global health. Psychol Health 2004;19:237–46.
22. John-Henderson N, Jacobs EG, Mendoza-Denton R, et al. Wealth, health and the moderating role of implicit social class bias. Ann Behav Med 2013;45:173–9.
23. Saxton KB, John-Henderson N, Reid M, et al. The social environment and IL-6 in rats and humans. Brain Behav Immun 2011;25:1617–25.
24. Rogers RG, Hummer RA, Nam CB. Living and dying in the USA: behavioral, health and social differential in adult mortality. San Diego (CA): Academic Press; 2000.
25. Clark R, Anderson NB, Clark VR, et al. Racism as a stressor for African Americans. A biopsychosocial model. Am Psychol 1999;54:805–16.
26. Ong AD, Fuller-Rowell T, Burrow AL. Racial discrimination and the stress process. J Pers Soc Psychol 2009;96:1259–71.
27. Borrell LN, Jacobs DR Jr, Williams DR, et al. Self reported racial discrimination and substance abuse in the Coronary Artery Risk Development in Adults study. Am J Epidemiol 2007;166:1068–79.
28. Kaszubowska L. Telomere shortening and ageing of the immune system. J Physiol Pharmacol 2008;59:169–86.
29. Saliques S, Zeller M, Lorin J, et al. Telomere length and cardiovascular disease. Arch Cardiovasc Dis 2010;103:454–9.
30. Valdes AM, Deary IJ, Gardner J, et al. Leukocyte telomere length is associated with cognitive performance in healthy women. Neurobiol Aging 2010;31:986–92.
31. Wolkowitz OM, Epel ES, Reus VI, et al. Depression gets old fast: do stress and depression accelerate cell aging? Depress Anxiety 2010;27:327–38.
32. Chae DH, Nuru-Jeter AM, Adler NE, et al. Discrimination, racial bias, and telomere length in African American men. Am J Prev Med 2014;46:103–11.
33. Health, United States, 2007 with chartbook on trends in the health of Americans. Hyattsville (MD): National Center for Health Statistics; 2007.
34. Brondolo E, Rieppi R, Kelly KP, et al. Perceived racism and blood pressure: a review of the literature and conceptual and methodological critique. Ann Behav Med 2003;25(1):55–65.
35. Chae DH, Nuru-Jeter AM, Adler NE. Implicit racial bias as a moderator of the association between racial discrimination and hypertension: a study of midlife African-American men. Psychosom Med 2012;74:961–4.
36. Latner JD, Stukard AJ. Getting worse: the stigmatization of obese children. Obes Res 2002;11:452–6.

37. Puhl R, Brownell KD. Obesity, bias and discrimination. Obes Res 2001;9: 788–805.
38. Muennig P. The body politic: the relationship between stigma and obesity-associated disease. BMC Public Health 2008;8:1–10.
39. Schupp HT, Brenner B. The implicit nature of the anti-fat bias. Front Hum Neurosci 2011;5:1–11.
40. Schwartz MB, Vartanian LR, Nosek BA, et al. The influence of one's own body weight on implicit and explicit anti-fat bias. Obesity 2006;14:440–7.
41. White AA III. Seeing patients: unconscious bias in health care. Cambridge (MA): Harvard University Press; 2011.
42. Chapman EN, Kaatz A, Carnes M. Physicians and implicit bias: how doctors may unwittingly perpetuate health disparities. J Gen Intern Med 2013;28:1504–10.
43. Sabin JA, Marini M, Nosek BA. Implicit and explicit anti-fat bias among a large sample of medical doctors by BMI, race, ethnicity and gender. PLoS one 2012; 7:e48448.
44. Sabin J, Nosek BA, Greenwald A, et al. Physicians' implicit and explicit attitudes about race by MD race, ethnicity and gender. J Health Care Poor Underserved 2009;20:896–913.
45. Cooper LA, Roter DL, Carson KA, et al. The associations of clinicians' implicit attitudes about race with medical visit communication and patient ratings of interpersonal care. Am J Public Health 2012;102:979–87.
46. Todd KH, Samaroo N, Hoffman JR. Ethnicity as a risk factor for inadequate emergency department analgesia. JAMA 1993;269:1537–9.
47. Todd KH, Deaton C, D'Adamo AP, et al. Ethnicity and analgesic practice. Ann Emerg Med 2000;35:11–6.
48. Todd KH, Lee T, Hoffman JR. The effect of ethnicity on physician estimates of pain severity in patients with isolated extremity trauma. JAMA 1994;271:925–8.
49. Green AR, Carney DR, Pallin DJ, et al. Implicit bias among physicians and its prediction of thrombolysis decisions for black and white patients. J Gen Intern Med 2007;22:1231–8.
50. Weitzman S, Cooper L, Chabless L, et al. Gender, racial and geographic differences in the performance of cardiac diagnostic and therapeutic procedures for hospitalized acute myocardial infarction in four states. Am J Cardiol 1997;79:722–6.
51. Blair IV, Steiner JF, Havranek EP. Unconscious (implicit) bias and health disparities: where do we go from here? Perm J 2011;15:71–8.
52. McEwen BS. Allostasis and allostatic load: implications for neuropsychopharmacology. Neuropsychopharmacology 2000;22:108–24.
53. Blair IV, Ma JE, Lenton AP. Imagining stereotypes away: the moderation of implicit stereotypes through mental imagery. J Pers Soc Psychol 2001;81:828–41.
54. Lowery BS, Hardin CD, Sinclair S. Social influence effects on automatic racial prejudice. J Pers Soc Psychol 2001;81:842–55.
55. Macrae CN, Bodenhausen GV, Milne AB, et al. Out of mind but back in sight. Stereotypes on the rebound. J Pers Soc Psychol 1994;67:808–17.
56. Richeson JA, Ambady N. Effects of situational power on automatic racial prejudice. J Exp Soc Psychol 2003;39:177–83.
57. Melek S, Norris D, Paulus J. Economic impact of integrated medicalbehavioral health: implications for psychiatry. Arlington (VA): American Psychiatric Association; 2013.
58. Blair IV, Havranek EP, Price DW, et al. Assessment of biases against Latinos and African Americans among primary care providers and community members. Am J Public Health 2013;103:92–8.

Child Soldiers

Children Associated with Fighting Forces

Suzan J. Song, MD, MPH, PhD(c)[a,b,*], Joop de Jong, MD, PhD[c,d]

KEYWORDS

• Child soldier • Trauma • War • Mental health • Gender-based violence

KEY POINTS

- Around the world, there are an estimated 300,000 to 500,000 children involved in armed conflict.
- Children can be abducted into a fighting force to fight or serve as sex slaves.
- Child soldiers have been shown to have depression, anxiety, and posttraumatic stress symptoms.
- Nongovernmental organizations, academic researchers, and clinicians have tried various mental health interventions, with promising results.
- Child and adolescent psychiatrists are uniquely trained in understanding and assisting youth to heal from having endured such extraordinary experiences.

INTRODUCTION

War and armed conflict have claimed the lives of 2 million children in the past decade.[1] Around the world, these wars and armed conflicts have included the conscription of children into armed forces. The term children associated with fighting forces has been used by many working in child protection, instead of the term child soldier, to better represent the diversity of children involved with fighting forces. For the sake of readability, this article uses the colloquial term child soldier or former child soldier to describe children associated with armed forces.

A child soldier is defined as someone "Below 18 years of age who is or has been recruited or used by an armed group in any capacity, including as fighters, cooks, porters, messengers, spies, or for sexual purposes. It does not refer only to a child

Financial disclosures: none.

[a] Department of Psychiatry, George Washington University School of Medicine, 2120 L Street, NW, Washington, DC 20037, USA; [b] Department of Psychiatry and Anthropology, Amsterdam Institute for Social Science Research (AISSR), University of Amsterdam, Amsterdam, The Netherlands; [c] Department of Psychiatry, VU University Medical Center, Amsterdam, AISSR, University of Amsterdam, Amsterdam, The Netherlands; [d] Department of Psychiatry, Boston University School of Medicine, Boston, MA, USA
* Corresponding author. 60 20th Street, 317, San Francisco, CA 94110.
E-mail address: suzan.song@post.harvard.edu

Child Adolesc Psychiatric Clin N Am 24 (2015) 765–775
http://dx.doi.org/10.1016/j.chc.2015.06.006 childpsych.theclinics.com
1056-4993/15/$ – see front matter

who is taking or has taken a direct part in hostilities."[2] Within this definition, it should be highlighted that child soldiers are not only those who use weapons to pillage villages and engage in mass rapes. In addition, so-called bush girls and boys have also been used for such purposes as human shields, mine sweepers, and guards. This knowledge has important implications for defining who receives services after a ceasefire.

Despite international regulations, in 2006 more than 250,000 children and adolescents were participants in armed forces around the world.[3] Child soldiering is not specific to any country or culture. Limited opportunities for healthy child development, unstable political security, poverty, and population displacement are all factors that can contribute to an environment in which children are not protected from joining the armed forces and are made vulnerable to be exploited. Rebel or terrorist groups may not abide by humanitarian law that protects civilians; therefore, the use of children in these settings can pose even greater risks to children in a war situation.

EXPERIENCE OF A CHILD SOLDIER

The first Global Report on Child Soldiers in 2001 showed that girls and boys were abducted into government forces and armed groups around the world.[4] Many children were forcibly recruited into the armed forces when villages, schools, and homes were raided. Families were threatened with death or severe punishment if the request to take the child was denied. Children as young as 7 years old were both abducted and recruited to fight in the armed forces, because they were thought to be easier to control and were considered to be fearless.[5]

Some countries, such as Sierra Leone and Mozambique, forced children to physically harm their families, kill a family member, or ransack their village, both to prevent them from having a place to come home to (the armed force becoming their new home) and to weaken or disrupt family ties that are often strong in interdependent societies. Often, abduction included witnessing extreme violence.[6] Some children reported joining the armed forces voluntarily; however, when joining was necessary for survival, or when there were few other opportunities for protection, it is unclear how voluntary this was. Some children joined out of revenge, because loved ones were brutally killed or humiliated because of their ethnic or religious affiliations. In many cultures that value ancestry, killing a family member may imply psychological suicide. The soul of the perpetrator becomes unable to be reincarnated, and hence remains in the nebulous space between life and death as a perpetual family outcast. Many believe that the soul could become a revengeful spirit attacking the living with misfortune.[7] Other children were reported to have joined for social inclusion, political ideology, to enter manhood precociously, or to escape exploitation (forced marriage) or abuse.[8] The initiation process of involvement in violence often takes place in steps, making it increasingly difficult for the children to extricate themselves.[9]

When a war ends and ceasefire ensues, the international community usually comes to assist in the process of reintegrating soldiers into civilian life. In many countries, such as Angola, Burundi, Liberia, Nepal, Mozambique, Uganda, and Sierra Leone, disarmament, demobilization, and reintegration (DDR) programs have been designed specifically to assist child soldiers to assimilate back into the civilian world. Disarmament involves soldiers showing that they know how to use weapons, then turning the weapons over. Demobilization then formally disbands the child soldier groups into the civilian world. The third phase is reintegration, in which child soldiers are then placed into the community, where they may face stigma and livelihood hardships with little economic or educational opportunities that could help meet basic needs. Some basic elements of reintegration programs consist of[10]:

- Interim care centers providing medical and psychosocial care
- Community discussions to sensitize the community about the return and the social inclusion of child soldiers
- Family tracing and reunification assistance
- Community-based systems of monitoring to assist
- Paying for school fees and training in vocational skills and income generation
- Conflict resolution and community sensitization

GENDER-BASED VIOLENCE

Girls also serve as child soldiers during armed combat, some as fighters, and others as cooks and sex slaves. Several reports suggest that they comprise almost 40% of child soldiers worldwide.[11] These experiences often lead to violence, unwanted pregnancies, and later to social stigmatization and abandonment. Many more girls experience severe psychosocial stress compared with the boy soldiers,[12] because sexual violence is more prevalent against girl soldiers[10,13,14] even though boys are vulnerable as well.[15] Kohrt and colleagues[16] reported that girls had lower confidence and prosocial behaviors, and were more likely to have posttraumatic stress disorder (PTSD) if they were soldiers, whereas boys were more likely to have PTSD if they were civilians.

Some girl soldiers are forced to have sexual relations with their chief/commanders, and are left with children as a product of rape. Some even give birth to children on the battlefield.[17] The infant can then become a burden for the girl soldier, who is left alone to care for the child, without financial or social support from the father. In some cases, as the girl soldier grows up, the child can remind her of her perpetrator, creating a strained relationship between mother and child.[15] Stigma against former girl soldiers can be increased for those who have experienced sexual violence, or who have children as a result of rape.[18,19] Being a survivor of sexual violence is taboo in many cultures, because of the notion that women are damaged, impure, or dirty, or the belief of many that the woman is to blame for being violated.[12,20] Not only do girls have the stigma of being raped, they also have the (self) stigma of being a former child soldier. In a study by Betancourt and colleagues,[21] girl soldiers had lower acceptance rates back into the community after the war was over, compared with boy soldiers. Moreover, some girl soldiers were excluded from the DDR programs at the end of the war, because many girls had not had fighter roles but had noncombat roles (cooks, porters, sex slaves). In many instances the aide community offers other services specifically for girl soldiers, in gender-based violence programs.[5]

MENTAL HEALTH OF FORMER CHILD SOLDIERS

Many researchers have studied the mental health of former child soldiers, although most studies use Western constructs of mental health (such as PTSD, depression, and anxiety). Because it is unclear whether these diagnostic frameworks are appropriate in the settings in which former child soldiers live, some researchers use dimensional scales to assess mental distress, or use qualitative interviews to define local mental health constructs.[22] The term cultural concept of distress (CCD) is a new addition to the Diagnostic and Statistical Manual of Mental Disorders, Fifth Edition, defined as "ways that cultural groups experience, understand, and communicate suffering, behavioral problems, or troubling thoughts and emotions."[23] They are described through (1) cultural syndromes, (2) idioms of distress, and (3) explanations.

Cultural syndromes are described as "clusters of symptoms and attributions that tend to co-occur among individuals in specific cultural groups, communities, or contexts, and that are recognized locally as coherent patterns of experience"[23]; cultural idioms of distress as "ways of expressing distress that may not involve specific symptoms or syndromes, but that provide collective, shared ways of experiencing and talking about personal or social concerns"[23] and (3) cultural explanations of distress or perceived causes as "labels, attributions, or features of an explanatory model that indicate culturally recognized meaning or etiology for symptoms, illness, or distress."[23] Kohrt and colleagues[24] (2013) argued that mental health intervention research should include both psychiatric outcomes and CCDs to ensure that culturally salient indicators of distress are addressed and resolved in treatment.

The literature is still growing, because many studies focus on cross-sectional data and do not have adequate comparison groups. An overview of some mental health studies of former child soldiers, along with longitudinal studies and studies with a comparison group, is provided later. A systematic review of mental health for former child soldiers found that only 10 of 21 studies used validated instruments for the local setting, and only 6 used multivariate approaches.[25] The review found that few studies assessed community and political factors influencing the child soldier experience; there were few scales validated for the local population, but, overall, children have chronic mental health problems after their experience as a child soldier, particularly if exposed to harsh violence and with reintegration stress of few family, community, and economic supports.[22]

When children as young as 7 years old are conscripted into the armed forces during wars that last for more than a decade (eg, Sierra Leone and Liberia), mental health and regular child development are greatly affected.[26] Case studies have shown that being a child in an armed group can lead to disruptions of autonomy, learning adult roles, and caretaking in later years, as well as trust.[23,27] Numerous studies in postconflict countries have shown the adverse mental health consequences of the child soldier experience, although there is large variability related to the differences in methodology of studies. Posttraumatic stress symptoms have been identified in former child soldiers in Uganda[12] and the Democratic Republic of Congo.[28] However, the PTSD rates range from 27%[29] to 97%,[12] or 99%[13] of a sample having PTSD symptoms. When compared, the prevalence of PTSD was higher among former child soldiers than never-conscripted children,[14,26] although other studies found little difference in mental distress between comparison groups.[30,31] Studies show that age of abduction did not have a strong association with postconflict reintegration, except for Betancourt and colleagues[12] (2010), who found that younger age of involvement predicted depressive symptoms.

Studies have also shown that former child soldiers have struggled not only with posttraumatic stress symptoms but general depression and anxiety symptoms as well.[14,18,32] After the war ends and child soldiers return to their homes, many think that they have few vocational skills and are overwhelmed with the stress of finding a job. Some child soldiers report sadness because they spent so many of their growing years in an armed force, when others their age were studying in school or learning other skills about how to work.[15,28] Moreover, child soldiers may feel guilty about their violent actions during the war. A study in Uganda showed that 51% of the former child soldiers perceived themselves as victims and 19% as perpetrators.[33]

Longitudinal Studies

Longitudinal studies can show the longer-term effects of child soldiering on mental health and functioning in youth. One 16-year longitudinal study in Mozambique collected qualitative data from 39 male former child soldiers and found they became productive and caring adults but continued to struggle with their war memories.[34] Betancourt and colleagues (2012)[31] conduced a 6-year longitudinal study of 259 former child soldiers and 127 self-integrated child soldiers in Sierra Leone and found high rates of depression, anxiety, and hostility, and these rates attenuated over time. Stigma against former child soldiers has been documented for those trying to reintegrate to their communities, who may be feared and marginalized by the community,[7,15,23,35] and this can be a prominent risk factor for mental distress. Longitudinal studies have emphasized several vulnerability and risk factors that have been found to be associated with poorer mental health outcomes in former child soldiers:

- Witnessing, experiencing, and perpetrating violence
- Young age of involvement
- Length of time in armed group
- Family abuse
- Neglect
- Stigma (leading to family and community rejection)
- Disappointment on return home
- Increased social disorder in the community
- Witnessed death of a family member or peer
- Exposure to torture
- Deprivation of food and water
- Being forced to perform rituals
- Killings
- Being a victim of sexual violence

Comparison Groups

When assessing mental health symptoms in the former child soldier population, a comparison group can help further differentiate between abnormal conditions and the general mental distress associated with war and armed conflict. Kohrt and colleagues (2008),[14] compared 141 former child soldiers in Nepal with 141 of their never-conscripted peers, and former child soldiers had more severe depression and PTSD than children never conscripted, even after controlling for trauma exposure. In a much smaller preliminary study by Song and colleagues[36] (2013) of 30 subjects from Burundi, there were no significant differences in mental health issues or aggression between former child soldiers and their gender-matched, age-matched, and village-matched civilian peers.[34]

Intergenerational Trauma

The first series of studies of intergenerational stress between former child soldiers and their children was a preliminary study comparing 15 male and female former child soldiers (now adults) with 15 never-conscripted civilian parents who were matched by age, gender, and village. Eleven children of former child soldiers and 9 children of civilians were also compared.[34] When former child soldiers (now adults) and civilian parents were compared, they had no significant difference in mental health problems. However, among their offspring, children of former child soldiers had significantly more conduct problems, worse coping skills, and felt less connected to community, siblings, and family.[34] A follow-up qualitative study of 40 adults (25 former child soldiers and 15 matched civilians) evaluated how intergenerational stress might be passed from former child soldiers to their children. The study found 3 main ways in which stress was transmitted: through parental discipline shaped by their rebel experience; severe parental emotional distress; and the community transmission of stress, including stigma.[15] The children of former child soldiers may have had more conduct problems because of the stigma that their parents faced, or if their parents had severe emotional distress that could have strained the parent-child relationship.

Protective Factors for Former Child Soldiers

Some factors have been shown to decrease the probability of having mental health problems. Family acceptance is a critical factor in improving the reintegration process for the former child soldiers back into their communities. In El Salvador, former child soldiers noted that family relationships were the most important factor that helped with reintegration.[30] Many child soldiers can leave the armed forces after the war and return to their home villages, where they may have pillaged or created harm during their recruitment/abduction process. These home communities can hold former child soldiers accountable for the destruction of the social fabric of their communities, and for the deaths or injuries caused to loved ones and neighbors. When child soldiers return, they are not always welcomed by the community. Those child soldiers who felt social support and community acceptance had more prosocial behaviors.[33] Research on former child soldiers in Nepal showed that family and community support predicted lower levels of mental distress and poor functioning. Being from a Buddhist minority ethnic group, being older, having a nuclear family, being abducted into an armed group, and not living in a high-caste society were associated with more social support.[19]

Educational opportunities for former child soldiers after the war are also important in the reintegration process. In general, school can provide an avenue for children to gain social and emotional development in addition to learning an academic curriculum. Because most child soldiers were not attending school, their socialization occurred in the armed group, with little opportunity for individual expression. Some former child soldiers reported multiple social difficulties that arose from their time in war. As child soldiers, they were not allowed to have friendships; to do so meant to put themselves and their friends in danger. If they made a mistake, such as talking out of turn, or were suspected of trying to escape, not only that child soldier but also anyone assumed to be a friend would be punished or killed.[15] Former child soldiers who were are able to return to school had more prosocial behaviors[12] and fewer mental health issues.[37] The years lost when children could have been pursuing education and economic opportunities can continue to be a major stressor for those who are no longer child soldiers. The basic life challenges that former child soldiers face after reintegration can be more difficult to manage than some of the experiences in the war. Despite these challenges, a large number of former child soldiers are able to survive through the war and be productive members of the community.

PSYCHOSOCIAL INTERVENTIONS FOR FORMER CHILD SOLDIERS

Because many armed conflicts that use child soldiers occur in low-income countries, there are few resources that are capable of managing the serious mental health needs of child soldiers returning to the community after a war.[38] These countries have few psychiatrists, psychologists, and other mental health professionals, and therefore communities are left seeking mental health care from their traditional healers, the religious community, or possibly the general physicians. With few professionals who have years of extensive training in mental health, a feasible plan for care would draw on community resources and local coping.[6] However, many mental health and psychosocial interventions for former child soldiers are provided by Westerners, and therefore are typically based on the Western notions of how to treat trauma: through the diagnosis and treatment of an individual.[39] A public mental health framework that includes prevention through treatment interventions would incorporate community, family, and social involvement.

Mental Health–focused Interventions

Clinical interventions should not only address the mental distress symptoms that former child soldiers may endure but also the impairment in functioning in society (eg, in school or in family and community responsibilities). Some former child soldiers experience severe mental health issues similar to depression, anxiety, and posttraumatic stress, which can affect relationships, parenting, and work. Interventions by the nongovernmental community typically focus on individual or group counseling. Because of the lack of available mental health professionals in many low-income/low-resource countries, longer-term, focused clinical interventions are typically not present.

Many studies report group-treatment models for war-affected youth, which may assist in scaling up services for those in need. An interventional study in northern Uganda on war-affected youth (with some former child soldiers) showed that group interpersonal therapy had more positive effects on depression in girls who were abducted than boys.[40] Short-term group crisis interventions have used the following modalities:

- Free play, storytelling, and drawing, to focus on a crisis period[41]
- Mind-body techniques[42]
- Dyadic mother-child therapy[43]
- School-based interventions[44]
- Trauma-focused/narrative exposure therapy[45]
- Supportive and cognitive-behavior therapy components[46]

Psychosocial Focused Interventions

Because several studies have shown that the social contexts of peer, family, and community are critical to former child soldiers,[47–48] interventions that include social and community factors are important in caring for this population. Community acceptance has been associated with adaptive attitudes and behaviors of former child soldiers, regardless of violence exposure.[12,33] Moreover, former child soldiers with lower exposure to current domestic violence had better family lives.[11] However, many psychosocial programs are found in unpublished manuals or internal nongovernmental organizational reports, with few undergoing rigorous evaluation. DDR programs can include community sensitization (in which noncombatants and former combatants join to discuss the reintegration process and facilitate communication). These programs are further enhanced and facilitated by family, education, vocational training, the payment of school fees, grants, and a myriad of reconciliation and skills programs. The Christian Children's Fund used a community empowerment approach with peace education and the United Nations Children's Fund (UNICEF) Community-based Reintegration Program established community-based child protection systems to provide educational and psychosocial support to former child soldiers.[49] Traditional healing practices are reported to be helpful in assisting the community acceptance of the child soldiers back into society. Cleansing ceremonies can represent community reconciliation by which former child soldiers can shed their contamination (for girl soldiers who were survivors of rape), and the community can show a willingness to reconcile.[50]

ROLE OF CHILD AND ADOLESCENT PSYCHIATRISTS

Skilled child and adolescent psychiatrists are uniquely positioned to understand the needs and strengths of children associated with armed forces. With an understanding of the biological, psychological, and social determinants of development and behavior, psychiatrists can integrate the effects of potential traumatic brain injuries, malnutrition, impaired child development, and medical complications with the normal and abnormal responses to extremely abnormal experiences. Child and adolescent psychiatrists can also emphasize and enhance awareness of the effects of social support (or lack thereof), education, and culture on the presentation and development of mental health issues. Child and adolescent psychiatrists take an ecological approach to human development[51] by integrating and paying attention to individual difficulties and inherent strengths, and the role of the family, school, and community; and take into account the wider sociopolitical contexts in which children are raised. Interventions have focused on mental health needs in general for former child soldiers, but little has been done for those with more severe needs. Child development is such that children with severe, chronic trauma may use and allocate their inner resources and strengths for survival instead of emotional growth, thereby hindering the development of emotion regulation skills and secure attachments and relationships.[52]

Global child and adolescent psychiatrists therefore weave the clinical, conceptual, and scientific treatments in the understanding of mental stress, and focus on the importance of children's rights, education, health, and social and community influences, which all play major roles in the well-being of all children worldwide. The dialogue around psychological issues for youth who have endured extraordinary circumstances will undoubtedly require an ethical approach,[53] strong understanding of the sociopolitical influences on each child's life, and flexibility in being able to integrate local ideology and means of healing with trials of interventions that have worked in similar communities and situations around the world. Child and adolescent psychiatrists are unique in that they can have a wide range of roles to affect child mental health, from direct treatment to the training of providers, as well as educating school and community workers as part of a public health approach.

REFERENCES

1. United Nations Childrens' Fund. State of the World's children. New York: UNICEF; 2007. Available at: http://www.unicef.org/publications/files/The_State_of_the_Worlds__Children__2007_e.pdf. Accessed December 7, 2014.
2. United Nations Children's Fund. Paris principles: principles and guidelines on children associated with armed forces or armed groups. p. 7. 2007. Available at: http://www.unicef.org/emerg/files/ParisPrinciples310107English.pdf. Accessed September 14, 2014.
3. Office of the Special Representative of the Secretary-General for Children and Armed Conflict (2006). Report to the General Assembly. A/61/275. 2006. Available at: http://www.un.org/children/conflict/english/reports.html. Accessed September 14, 2014.
4. The Coalition to Stop the Use of Child Soldiers. Child soldiers global report 2004. London: Coalition to Stop the Use of Child Soldiers; 2004.
5. The Coalition to Stop the Use of Child Soldiers. Democratic Republic of the Congo: priorities for children associated with armed forces and groups. London: Coalition to Stop the Use of Child Soldiers; 2007.
6. Wessells MG, Monteiro C. Healing the wounds following protracted conflict in Angola: a community-based approach to assisting war-affected children.

In: Gielen UP, Fish J, Draguns JG, editors. Handbook of culture, therapy, and healing. Mahwah (NJ): Erlbaum; 2004. p. 321–41.
7. De Jong J. Public mental health in socio-cultural context. In: de Jong J, editor. Trauma, war, and violence. New York: Plenum Publishers; 2002. p. 454.
8. Wessells M. Child soldiering: entry, reintegration, and breaking cycles of violence. In: Fitzduff M, Stout C, editors. The psychology of resolving global conflicts: from war to peace. Westport (CT): Praeger Security International; 2006. p. 243–66.
9. Vines A. Renamo terrorism in Mozambique. Bloomington (IN): Indiana University Press; 1991.
10. Verhey B. Child soldiers: preventing, demobilizing and reintegrating. Africa region working paper series. Washington, DC: World Bank; 2001. p. 15–21. Available at: http://www.worldbank.org/afr/wps/wp23.pdf.
11. McKay S, Mazurana D. Where are the girls? Girls in fighting forces in Northern Uganda, Sierra Leone, and Mozambique: their lives during and after war. Montreal (Canada): International Center for Human Rights and Democratic Development; 2004. p. 1–146.
12. Betancourt TS, Borisova I, de la Soudiere M, et al. Sierra Leone's child soldiers: war exposures and mental health problems by gender. J Adolesc Health 2011;49: 21–8.
13. Klasen F, Oettingen G, Daniels J, et al. Posttraumatic resilience in former child soldiers. Child Dev 2010;81(4):1096–113.
14. Bayer CP, Klasen F, Adam H. Association of trauma and PTSD symptoms with openness to reconciliation and feelings of revenge among former Ugandan and Congolese child soldiers. J Am Med Assoc 2007;298(5):555–9.
15. Amone P'Olak K, Garnefski N, Kraaij V. The impact of war experiences and physical abuse on formerly abducted boys in northern Uganda. S Afr Psychiatr Rev 2007;10:76–82.
16. Kohrt B, Jordans M, Tol WA, et al. Comparison of mental health between ex child soldiers and children never conscripted by armed groups in Nepal. J Am Med Assoc 2008;300(6):691–702.
17. Song SJ, Tol WA, de Jong J. Indero: intergenerational trauma and resilience between Burundian former child soldiers and their children. Fam Process 2014; 53(2):239–51.
18. Coulter C, Persson M, Utas M. Young female fighters in African wars: conflict and its consequences. The Nordic Africa Institute; 2008. Policy Dialogue No. 3. Available at: http://www.gsdrc.org/go/display&type=Document&id=3543. Accessed September 14, 2014.
19. Mazurana D, McKay S. Girls in fighting forces in Northern Uganda, Sierra Leone, and Mozambique: policy and program recommendations. United Nations Disarmament, Demobilization and Reintegration Resource Center; 2003. Available at: http://unddr.org/docs/Girls_in_Fighting_Forces.pdf. Accessed September 14, 2014.
20. Kohrt BA, Jordans MJ, Tol WA, et al. Social ecology of child soldiers: child, family, and community determinants of mental health, psychosocial well-being, and reintegration in Nepal. Transcult Psychiatry 2010;47:727–53.
21. Betancourt TS, Borisova I, Brennan RB, et al. Sierra Leone's former child soldiers: a follow-up study of psychosocial adjustment and community reintegration. Child Dev 2010;81(4):1077–95.
22. Bolton P, Tol WA, Bass J. Introduction to special issue: combining qualitative and quantitative research methods to support psychosocial and mental health programmes. Intervention 2009;7(3):181–6.

23. American Psychiatric Association. Diagnostic and statistical manual of mental disorders. 5th edition. Washington, DC: Author; 2013.
24. Kohrt BA, Rasmussen A, Kaiser BN, et al. Cultural concepts of distress and psychiatric disorders: literature review and research recommendations for global mental health epidemiology. Int J Epidemiol 2013;43:1–42.
25. Betancourt TS, Borisov I, Williams T, et al. Psychosocial adjustment and mental health in former child soldiers – a systematic review of the literature and recommendations for future research. J Child Psychol Psychiatry 2013;54(1):17–36.
26. Machel G. The impact of war on children. London: Hurst; 2001.
27. Song SJ, de Jong J. The role of silence in Burundian former child soldiers. Int J Adv Couns 2014;36(1):84.
28. Derulyn I, Broekaert E, Schuyten G, et al. Post-traumatic stress in ex Ugandan child soldiers. Lancet 2004;363(9412):861–3.
29. Okello J, Onen T, Musisi S. Psychiatric disorders among war-abducted and non-abducted adolescents in Gulu district, Uganda: a comparative study. Afr J Psychiatry 2007;20:225–31.
30. Blattman C, Annan J. The consequences of child soldiering. Rev Econ Stat 2010; 92:882–98.
31. Betancourt TS, McBain R, Newnham EA, et al. Trajectories of internalizing problems in war-affected Sierra Leonean youth: examining conflict and post-conflict factors. Child Dev 2012;84(2):455–70.
32. Santacruz ML, Arana RE. Experiences and psychosocial impact of the El Salvador civil war on child soldiers. Biomedica 2002;22(Suppl 2):383–97.
33. Klasen F, Reissmann S, Voss C, et al. The guiltless guilty: trauma-related guilt and psychopathology in former Ugandan child soldiers. Child Psychiatry Hum Dev 2015;46(2):180–93.
34. Boothby N, Crawford J, Halperin J. Mozambique child soldier life outcome study: lessons learned in rehabilitation and reintegration efforts. Glob Public Health 2006;1(1):87–107.
35. Betancourt TS, Agnew-Blias J, Gilman S, et al. Past horrors, present struggles: the role of stigma in the association between war experiences and psychosocial adjustment among former child soldiers in Sierra Leone. Soc Sci Med 2010;70:17–26.
36. Song SJ, de Jong J, O'Hara R, et al. Children of former child soldiers and never-conscripted civilians: a preliminary intergenerational study in Burundi. J Aggress Maltreat Trauma 2013;22(7):757.
37. Ovuga E, Oyok TO, Moro EB. Post traumatic stress disorder among former child soldiers attending a rehabilitative service and primary school education in northern Uganda. Afr Health Sci 2008;8:136–41.
38. Song SJ, van den Brink H, de Jong J. Who cares for former child soldiers? Mental health systems of care in Sierra Leone. Community Ment Health J 2013;49(5): 615–24.
39. Miller K, Rasco L. The mental health of refugees. Ecological approaches to healing and adaptation. Mahwah (NJ): Lawrence Erlbaum Associates; 2004.
40. Bolton P, Bass J, Betancourt T, et al. Interventions for depression symptoms among adolescent survivors of war and displacement in northern Uganda: a randomized controlled trial. J Am Med Assoc 2007;298(5):519–27.
41. Thabet A, Vostanis P. Post traumatic stress disorder reactions in children of war: a longitudinal study. Child Abuse Negl 2000;24(2):289–90.
42. Gordon JS, Staples JK, Blyta A, et al. Treatment of posttraumatic stress disorder in postwar Kosovo high school students using mind-body skills groups: a pilot study. J Trauma Stress 2004;17(2):143–7.

43. Dybdahl R. Children and mothers in war: an outcome study of a psychosocial intervention program. Child Dev 2001;72(4):1214–30.
44. Tol WA, Komproe I, Jordans M, et al. Outcomes and moderators of a preventive school-based mental health intervention for children affected by war in Sri Lanka: a cluster randomized trial. World Psychiatry 2012;11(2):114–22.
45. Onyut LP, Neuner F, Schauer E, et al. Narrative exposure therapy as a treatment for child war survivors with posttraumatic stress disorder: two case reports and a pilot study in an African refugee settlement. BMC Psychiatry 2005;5:7.
46. Stepakoff S, Hubbard J, Katoh M, et al. Trauma healing in refugee camps in Guinea: a psychosocial program for Liberian and Sierra Leonean survivors of torture and war. Am Psychol 2006;61(8):921–32.
47. Barber B. Political violence, social integration, and youth functioning: Palestinian youth from the Intifada. J Community Psychol 2001;29(3):259–80.
48. Prothrow-Stith D. Deadly consequences. New York: Harper & Collins Press; 1991.
49. Betancourt TS, Borisova I, Rubin-Smith JE, et al. Psychosocial adjustment and social reintegration of children associated with armed forces and armed groups: The state of the field and future directions. Austin, TX: Psychology Beyond Borders; 2008.
50. Stark L. Cleansing the wounds of war: an examination of traditional healing, psychosocial health and reintegration in Sierra Leone. Intervention 2006;4(3):206–18.
51. Bronfenbrenner U. The ecology of human development: experiments by nature and design. Cambridge (MA): Harvard University Press; 1979.
52. Van der Kolk BA. Developmental trauma disorder. Towards a rational diagnosis for chronically traumatized children. Psychiatr Ann 2005;35:401–8.
53. Song SJ. An ethical approach to lifelong learning: implications for global psychiatry. Acad Psychiatry 2011;35(6):391–6.

Challenges in Providing Child and Adolescent Psychiatric Services in Low Resource Countries

Savita Malhotra, MD, PhD*, Susanta Kumar Padhy, MD

KEYWORDS

• Child • Adolescent • Psychiatry • Challenges • Low and middle income countries

KEY POINTS

- Ninety percent of the world's children and adolescents live in low-income countries and about half of lifetime mental disorders begin before age 14.
- Specific national-level child and adolescent mental health (CAMH) policies, standardized service and training are virtually nonexistent; resources are insufficient, inequitably distributed, and inefficiently used; majority lack access to care.
- CAMH care has the potential to reduce psychiatric morbidity, enhance productivity, resilience and educational attainment.
- CAMH must be prioritized in the developmental and health agenda of countries.
- There is need to strengthen the capacity building by supplemental training by using innovative technologies like telepsychiatry, and mobile health technology.
- Establishing a network of services, formulating a national-level CAMH policy, generating funds for research, and creating more academic institutes providing superspecialty courses in child and adolescent psychiatry are immediate needs.

Low-resource countries comprise low- and middle-income countries (LAMIC), where not only are the resources scarce, but where the probability of extreme hardships and vulnerability to develop mental disorders is also greater.[1] One-third of the world's population comprises children and adolescents, and 90% of them live in LAMIC where they constitute up to 50% of the population.[2] Nearly one-half of all lifetime mental disorders begin before the age of 14 years.[3,4] The prevalence rates for child and adolescent mental disorders are around 20% worldwide, including in low-resource

Disclosures: None.
Child and Adolescent Psychiatry Unit, Department of Psychiatry, Postgraduate Institute of Medical Education and Research (PGIMER), Sector 12, Chandigarh 160012, India
* Corresponding author.
E-mail address: savita.pgi@gmail.com

Child Adolesc Psychiatric Clin N Am 24 (2015) 777–797
http://dx.doi.org/10.1016/j.chc.2015.06.007 childpsych.theclinics.com
1056-4993/15/$ – see front matter

countries.[5–7] Neuropsychiatric disorders account for 15% to 30% of the disability-adjusted life-years lost in the first 3 decades of life, of which the first 2 constitute childhood and adolescence.[8] In LAMIC, the median 1-year treated prevalence for children and adolescents is 4.2 times lower than that for the adult population.[8] This means that roughly fewer than 25% of children and adolescents with psychiatric disorders are treated compared with the proportion of adults with psychiatric illness who are treated in the LAMIC.

AVAILABILITY OF SERVICES

Resources

The world regions with the highest percentage of the population under the age of 19 years in LAMIC have the poorest level of resources.[4] Children and adolescents make up 12% of the patient population in mental health outpatient facilities and less than 6% in all other types of mental health facilities. Fewer than 1% of beds in inpatient facilities are reserved for children and adolescents.[8] The child ATLAS project (2005) documented that there are no pediatric beds for mental health in general hospitals/adult psychiatric facilities in low-income countries.[7] It is preferable to treat children and adolescents in the least restrictive environment as close to their community as possible, which requires a range of community-based services to provide a "continuum" of care from inpatient settings to outpatient care.[7,9] Developing a mechanism to provide a range of community services in this regard is not an easy task. Overall, there is a scarcity of resources for child and adolescent psychiatric services both at the hospital level as well as the community level. Very few nongovernment organizations (NGOs) focus on treatment, prevention, promotion, or policy development for children and adolescent psychiatric disorders, regardless of the income status of the country (majority focus on advocacy).[7] In most of the African, Eastern Mediterranean, Southeast Asian, and Western Pacific regions, the ratio of child psychiatrists to the population is 1 per 4 to 5 million. In less than one-third of all the countries worldwide, there is an identifiable institution or government office/entity responsible for child and adolescent mental health services (CAMH) services.[4,7–11]

There is a massive shortage of child and adolescent psychiatrists in low-resource countries, with more than 95% of specialized human resources concentrated in high-income countries.[1,7,9,11] There is little or no formal training imparted to behavioral and developmental pediatricians, general pediatricians, general psychiatrists, speech and language therapists, and other medical professionals involved in child and adolescent mental health.[1] Across low-resource countries, standards for training are absent, potential resources for CAMH are not used adequately, and supplemental training for the professional and paraprofessionals involved in the care of children and adolescents are not being implemented.[7,9] Training provided for mental health professionals in child and adolescent mental health is minimal, with fewer than 1% receiving some refresher training. Most countries (76%) organize educational activities on child and adolescent mental health.[8]

Research

Research on CAMH from LAMIC is meager, comprising only 3% to 6% of all published mental health research in the world. The proportion of psychiatrists in a country has a direct reflection on that country's research output.[12,13] Among the 670 randomized clinical trials (published in journals indexed in PubMed) on interventions for selected mental health problems in children and adolescents, only 58 came from middle-income countries and only one from a low-income country. There was lack of evidence of the efficacy of psychosocial or combined interventions and no effectiveness or cost-effectiveness trials.[14–16] The number of well-designed, methodologically sound studies are negligible in resource-poor countries.[15–20]

To Summarize

Resources are insufficient, inequitably distributed, and inefficiently used, resulting in a great majority of children and adolescents with mental disorder not receiving care at all. Even when available, treatment and care are often neither evidence based nor of high quality, resulting in a large treatment gap of more than 90% in many LAMIC countries.[6,21,22] To address this issue, the World Health Organization (WHO) launched the Mental Health Action Programme for high-priority conditions (based on larger burden in terms of morbidity, greater economic costs, and often associated with violation of human rights) that includes children and adolescents with mental disorders.[23]

CONCEPT OF EFFECTIVE CHILD AND ADOLESCENT MENTAL HEALTH SERVICES

Delivering CAMH requires a (1) thorough and comprehensive understanding of the developmental psychopathology and evolution of the child and adolescent mental disorders that may arise at any stage of development, such as periconception to perinatal to preschool, and school to adolescent periods; (2) involvement of professionals who might be needed to take care of the child during these periods, including obstetricians, pediatricians, general psychiatrists, child and adolescent psychiatrists, addiction specialists, social workers, physiotherapists, occupational therapists, psychiatric nurses, neurologists, school teachers, school counsellors, psychologists, speech and language therapists, special educators, behavior therapists, the criminal justice system, human right activists, and policy makers without underestimating the active role of the child and his or her family; and (3) immense intersectoral coordination and collaboration (**Fig. 1**). It is important to understand that providing CAMH services is heavily dependent on training and policy issues in the country (**Fig. 2**). It is necessary to keep in mind the cultural norms that the professionals have to work within. Services ought to be affordable, easily accessible, and cost effective to maintain the continuity of care and should be promotive and preventive in scope.

It is evident that policy, training, services, and research have complex and interdependent relationships whereby 1 influences the other in a reciprocal manner.

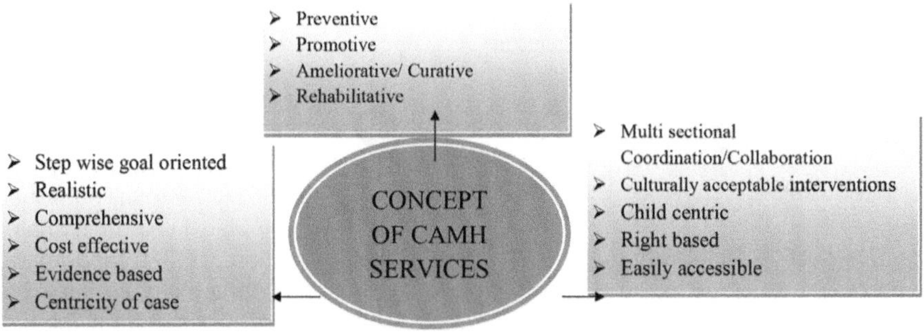

Fig. 1. Effective child and adolescent mental health (CAMH) services.

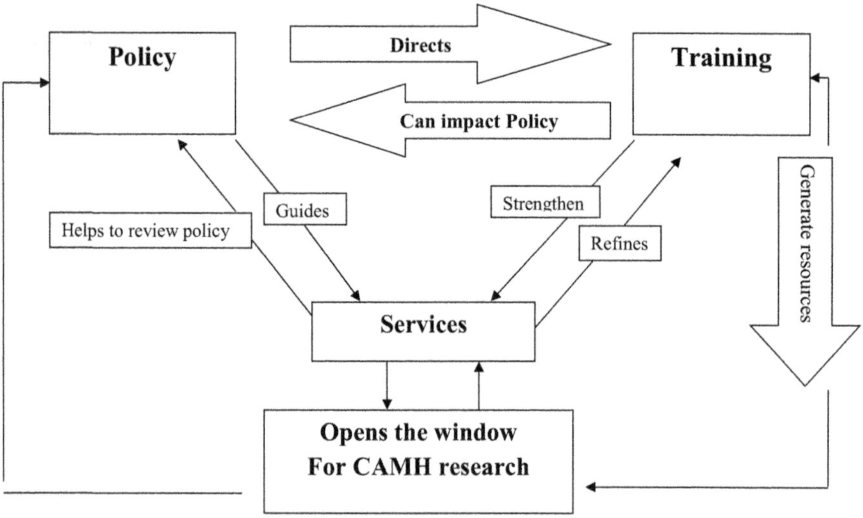

Fig. 2. Complex and interdependent relationship of policy, training, research, and services. CAMH, child and adolescent mental health.

Epidemiology

Epidemiologic studies starting from case identification to case management are a challenging task (**Fig. 3**). It is more so in the child and adolescent mental disorders because it is fraught with problems of interpretation of symptoms, cultural concepts of what constitutes abnormality,[24,25] inadequate reporting,[4,7] variation in definition, and when to consult a child and adolescent mental health professional. Problems are further compounded by limited access to medical services, and poor recognition of the early signs of neurodevelopmental or neurobehavioral disorders by the parents with socioeconomic disadvantage, or by day care centers/school teachers.[26] Methodologic differences among studies are another major source of difficulties in prevalence rates.[24]

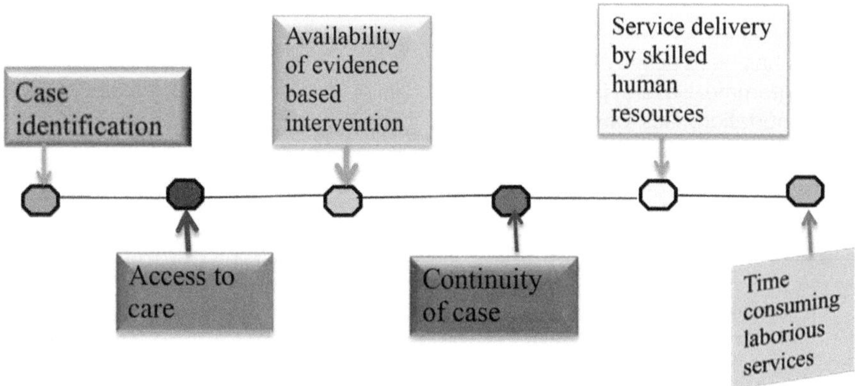

Fig. 3. Challenges in epidemiology.

Epidemiologic research relies on the use of valid and reliable assessment tools that are applicable to a given culture or population. For example, the Rutter's B scale for teachers, when applied to a representative sample of 963 Indian school children between the ages of 4 and 11 years at the recommended cutoff score of 9, had low sensitivity (51.8%) and very low specificity (34.1%).[27] Studies using only a screening instrument tended to yield greater prevalence rates, whereas those using detailed assessment tools to diagnose psychiatric disorders yielded lower prevalence rates.[28–30] Greater prevalence was also observed in countries with ongoing conflicts or war conditions[31] and is supported by a study conducted in SriLanka[32] done during the period of "ethnic crisis." A systematic review and metaregression analysis of 102 studies, attributed significant worldwide variability of prevalence of attention deficit hyperactivity disorder to methodologic differences. Geographic location was associated with significant variability only between estimates of attention deficit hyperactivity disorder from North America and both Africa and the Middle East.[28] However, youth's self-reported problems in 24 very different countries (n = 27,206), using multiple epidemiologic approaches were largely consistent.[29,30]

The difficulties in measuring the magnitude of the gap in CAMH include the following[8,9]: the capacity to gather consistent, meaningful epidemiologic data, which are largely absent in developing countries and the lack of an agreed framework for considering impairment. For example, 2 children with the same diagnosis can have markedly different degrees of impairment depending on family support, culture, and other factors. Therefore, assessing impairment in children and adolescents is a complex task and is relevant to the context.[33–37] In addition, the complexity of identifying the full range of services that might be helpful to an affected child creates difficulties. Children with mental health problems are often seen first and treated in the education, social service, or juvenile justice systems[38] and, therefore, may or may not be recorded as having mental health problems or needs. Further, some programs are targeted to specific problems and come under the sponsorship of NGOs, which often deliver services independent of government oversight.[9,13]

The labeling and understanding of child and adolescent mental disorders in the context of changing norms of the society makes the task even more complex. For example, in India, prevalence and distribution of eating disorders are begin altered[39] because of changing norms of "body image idealness" and "body weight ideal," which are largely driven by Western influence and/or media.[40,41]

IMPROVING ACCESS TO CARE

The vast majority of children in low-resource countries do not have access to care and this lack has been acknowledged as a major challenge in the WHO Mental Health Action Programme. Several factors that serve as barriers for accessing care include lack of transportation, lack of available treatment resources, limited financial resources, lack of ability to communicate effectively in the patient's language, and social stigma (37.5% in LIC vs 80% in high-income countries).[4,7] Patel and colleagues[1] in 2013 observed 3 major barriers in LAMIC: low resources, low detection of child and adolescent mental disorders, and lack of evidence on the delivery of treatments. Using screening measures for detection of probable disorders, coupled with a second stage diagnostic assessment is likely to improve detection. After detection, nonspecialist workers in community and school settings can be used for the delivery of psychosocial interventions. Existing human resources can be empowered with innovative technologies like telepsychiatry,[42] a mobile health technology.[1,43] This innovation is likely to be supported by increased availability of mobile phones, computers, and access to the Internet in LIC. A telepsychiatry model has been developed recently in India and has been used for direct patient care (diagnosis and management), consultation, training, education, and research purposes.[42,44] Both real-time, live interaction (synchronous) and store-forward (asynchronous) types of technologies have been used for these purposes. The local government in some states of India has distributed laptops, mobile telephones, bicycles free of cost to the school, and rural female students attending college to encourage and motivate them to continue their education. These gadgets can very well be used without any extra financial burden on the consumer or stakeholder for the purpose of sensitizing the children and adolescents about mental health issues, identifying high-risk groups for universal or selectively indicated prevention measures, developing support group among peers, crisis intervention helplines, and early identification of cases. Such mechanisms of care will also be suitable for continuum of care (ie, periodic follow-up) without much difficulty. The use of such electronic mechanisms can help to facilitate group education and interventions. In some instances, the use of these mechanisms can compensate also clearly for the shortage of skilled human resources, or the high work load and consequent burnout among existing child and adolescent mental health professionals in low-resource countries. In addition, health care resource use may also decrease. However, for this to be feasible and implementable, regional and national leaders (professionals and paraprofessionals working in the areas of child mental health and related areas including school personnel, volunteers, social workers, etc) must make a commitment, while portraying optimism and dedication. While devising such innovative mechanisms, one has to prioritize the conditions for which identification and interventions are to be made, keeping in mind cultural factors of the target population.

IDENTIFICATION OF THOSE IN NEED

A multicountry study across 9 countries (predominantly LAMIC) has demonstrated that providing adequate knowledge about mental health problems to parents, teachers, and students resulted in improved awareness about and detection of mental disorders in school children.[33] Media (electronic and print) has an important role to play in increasing the knowledge, and assessing the attitude, perception, and behavior of members of society including children and adolescents.[40] Media in some form or other (eg, radio, local newspaper) has a reach in the remotest area of low resource countries that can be of help in this regard.

In a study conducted in India, parents of 37.5% of children screened to have mental health problems felt the need to seek treatment.[35] In contrast, in a study in Korea the parents of 10.4% of school children perceived a need regarding mental health services for their children; and out of these, only 1.92% actually used mental health services.[36] Understanding the parents' recognition of their children's mental health issues and need for treatment is very important. Equally important is the parental threshold for reporting abnormal behaviors.[45,46]

An effective, low-cost method could be identification of conditions that are apparent and do not require sophisticated training, such as children with visual, hearing, and physical impairments.[1] Alternatively, screening questionnaires that are useful can be applied by trained community health workers followed by a second assessment by health professionals. Some of these questionnaires are the 39-item Neurodevelopmental Disorders Screening Questionnaire for identification of 10 neurodevelopmental disorders,[47] the Comprehensive Psychopathology Measurement Schedule, the Strengths and Difficult Questionnaire (www.sdqinfo.com), and The Child Behavior Check list. The Comprehensive Psychopathology Measurement Schedule has an

Indian version that has been adapted.[47] These 2 strategies, when coordinated with school-based and clinic-based services, are likely to improve early identification of children and adolescents who need intervention.

In low-resource countries, the number of street children (whether homeless, addicts, or victims of sexual abuse or trafficking) is disproportionately high and there are no adequate homes or institutions for them in comparison with high-income countries. These children are at increased risk for the development of child and adolescent mental health disorders. The Equilibrium Project in Sao Paulo, Brazil, is an example where child psychiatrists from a university setting have taken to the streets and developed a partnership with the children and adolescents on the streets.[48] The regions that are prone to war, conflict, and natural disaster are likely to have more CAMH morbidity and should develop services for early identification of cases. Research aiming to improve access to care for child and adolescent mental disorders has emerged as one of the leading challenges in global mental health.[49]

Interventions

Interventions for child and adolescent mental health disorders should include health promotion, prevention, and treatment. Child mental health promotion and prevention should take into account all of the risk, protective and promotive factors. Such risk and protective factors can be present "within the child" (eg, temperament or intelligence) or in the "environment."[13] There is a complex interplay of individual determinants with the family and sociocultural determinants of mental disorders provides the backdrop upon which promotive and preventive services for children and adolescents are based.[11,13] **Fig. 4** illustrates this interaction.

A study in Brazilian schoolchildren aged 7 to 14 years showed that childhood psychopathology was independently associated with living in a dangerous area, a nontraditional family system, parental stress, harsh physical punishment, poor general health, low IQ, repeating a school grade, and male gender.[50] Seizure disorders and brain infections in childhood, which are more common in many LAMIC, are also associated strongly with behavior and emotional disorders.[51,52] There is consistent evidence that authoritative parenting is a robust protective factor for the development of psychopathology and positive adjustment among adolescents.[53] The authors of this article have described strategies for CAMH promotion focusing on building capacity in children and adolescents, in parents and families, in the school and health systems, and in the wider community, including structural interventions; and on wider public health strategies for prevention and promotion. In particular, capacity needs to be built across the health system focusing on low-cost, universally available and accessible resources, and on empowering families and children. We also consider the role of formal teaching and training programs, and the role for specialists in CAMH promotion.[13]

Focusing on positive mental health will not only decrease the burden of child and adolescent mental health disorders but will also enhance the socioeconomic indices of the country and vice-versa. We present 2 examples to substantiate this supposition.

Example 1

A study from China showed that children who are left behind in school had significantly more psychopathology and less prosocial behaviors on the Strength and Difficulties Questionnaire than those who had no history of having been left behind.[54] A 2-stage Malaysian study and a study done in Turkey also reported a greater prevalence of emotional and behavioral disorders in this subset of population.[55,56] Children and adolescents with behavioral and emotional problems, such as oppositional behaviors,

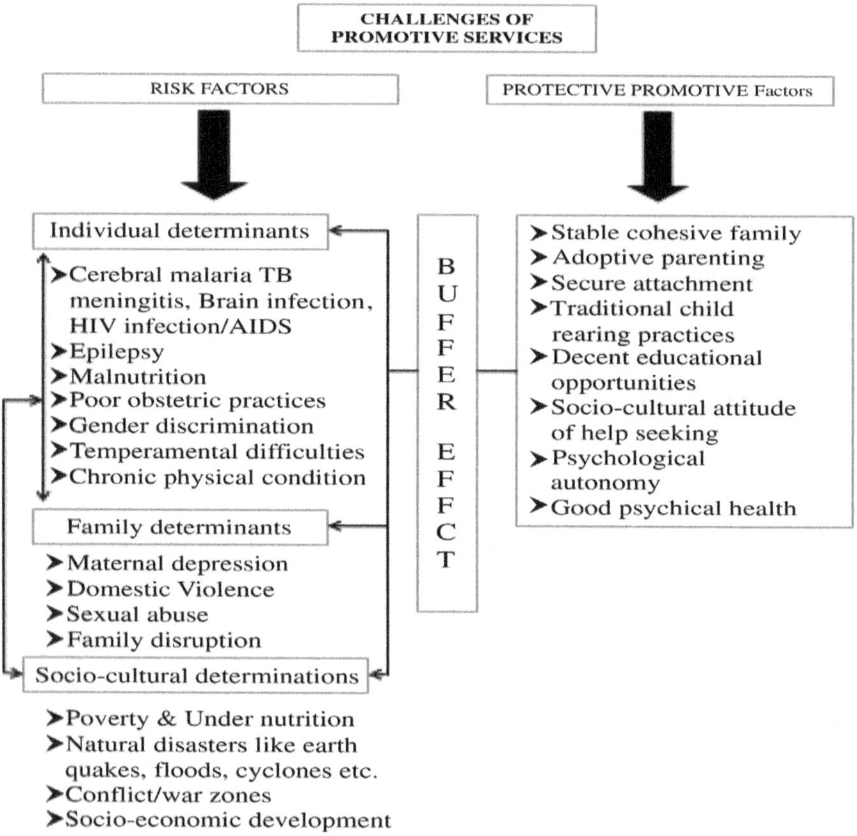

Fig. 4. Complex interaction of risk and protective factors relevant to child and adolescent mental health. HIV, human immunodeficiency virus.

conduct disorder, substance use/abuse, specific learning disorders, baseline intellectual disabilities, brain damage, sensory/motor deficits, lack of educational preparation, and psychosocial disturbances, help to contribute to a lower level of educational attainment and with early and appropriate interventions can improve their educational attainment. It is well-known that children dropping out of school is less likely to occur when the causes are prevented, addressed, and treated early.[57–60] A recent cluster trial in preschools in Jamaica described the benefits of a low-cost, school-based intervention, delivered by teachers, reduced child conduct problems and increased child social skills at home and at school.[34] However, teachers, particularly in primary and secondary schools, are already struggling with systemic challenges, like overcrowded class rooms, inadequate resources, inconsistent quality and low teacher to student ratio.[61] Taking on yet another task can compromise the routine responsibility of formal teaching.[33]

Example 2

Maternal depression during pregnancy and after child birth is associated with impaired development of attachment, cognition, language, developmental milestones, and can lead to childhood undernutrition and stunting.[62] It can also lead to low birth weight, premature birth, and other obstetric complications that are more common in LAMIC countries. Nearly 20% of all pregnancies in LAMIC countries occur in women under the age of 19 years and are associated with adverse maternal and child outcomes. Such obstetric complications in turn hamper healthy development of the child, further adding to the risk of developing child and adolescent mental health problems.

According to the authors, the real challenge would be to find strategies for the individual risk, promotive, and protective factors. Ideally these should be in order of priority as per prevalence and the impact of such factors, on a given nation or region of a particular country. Some of these strategies are already available at a systemic level. For example in India, a successful program has already been put into place: The Reproductive and Child Health (I and II) Program to take care of the antenatal and postnatal checkups, monitoring of pregnant mothers; assessment of the nutritional status of the child and immunization status of the child, and so on. However, the promotion of positive mental health, identification of risk and protective factors in the mother, child, and family, and early identification of mental health issues of children and adolescents has not been given due importance. Because developing and implementing a new program in low resource countries can be a difficult task, a feasible solution is the strengthening of an already existing successful program (eg, the Reproductive and Child Health program in India). This helps to sensitize health care workers to mental health issues by providing supplemental training.

Studies from India, China, and Brazil, as well as other countries have demonstrated the buffering effect of authoritarian and sensitive parenting, a strong family system, faith in religion and belief in destiny, traditional prescriptions of hierarchy, and a positive role of grandparents in child rearing.[13,24,50,53,63–67]

Many LAMIC, including India, are undergoing societal transition in the form of altered sex ratio, changing family structure and family dynamics, changing gender roles, an increased proportion of working mothers, increasing sexual abuse and domestic violence, and urbanization.[30,50,63,68–70] Studies from India[63] and cross-cultural studies from Asian communities,[50,70] Brazil,[50] South Africa[71] have shown that enmeshed family structure and family functioning, unhealthy parenting styles like insensitive parenting, negative sociocultural attitude toward relationship and family, partner violence increases the risk of childhood psychopathology and child and adolescent mental disorders.[13] Therefore, there is an urgent need for all stakeholders in child and adolescent mental health to address these issues of social transition in a more balanced and acceptable manner to minimize the risk it may have on the children's mental health. Child and adolescent mental health professionals can help to sensitize communities to the impact of social factors on mental health of children.

One has to move forward from promotive to preventive services. Although there is good evidence for efficacy and cost-effective interventions in some specific child adolescent mental disorders, a very small number of such interventions have been evaluated in LAMIC countries.[72–75] An evidence base for low-cost, community-based interventions for children in LAMIC is lacking.[72–75] A systematic review on evidence and treatment approaches for children affected by war in LAMIC by Jordans and colleagues[74] found a moderate effect size for treatment efficacy but were found to be largely the results of within-group change rather than an effect of treatment. Overall, there is a general lack of empirical evidence for interventions.[72,75]

Some programs already running in LAMIC countries are a step toward low cost interventions at the community level. Some of them are: Integrated Child Development Scheme in India,[76] the PANDAI (Child Development and Mother's Care) Project in Indonesia,[77] the PRONOEI program in Peru,[78] the PROAPE program in Brazil, the Integrated Program for Child and Family Development in Thailand,[79] and the *Hogares Comunitarios de Bienestar* program in Colombia.[80] All of these programs target children younger than 7 years of age, and implemented mainly with low-cost, basic health workers recruited from the local community focusing on malnutrition, promoting psychosocial development, parenting, and preschool educational interventions, immunization, and support for mothers.

As a step toward capacity building Brazil, for example, has designed specialized services such as CAPSi (Psychosocial Community Care Center for Children and Adolescents) to assist severe cases and further development of both primary care and specialized (beyond the CAPSi model) services, creating different levels of care by enhancing partnership within and outside the health sector. The presence of the Guardianship Councils, CAPSi, ESF (Estratégia de Saúde da Família), and NASF (Núcleo de Apoio à Saúde da Família) provide much of the necessary framework for the expansion of responsive, quality care for children and adolescents with mental disorders.

Financial and career development incentives could be important drivers to motivate employment seeking in the public health system.[81]

These intervention services to be delivered need an effective capacity building process (**Fig. 5**) in place. The points that are important and to be kept in mind during the building process are (1) developing an ethos of broad understanding of holistic, comprehensive positive mental health well-being, and not merely an absence of a child and adolescent mental disorder, (2) setting prioritized and realistic achievable goals, (3) focusing on low-cost community resources at different levels of health and education system, and (4) targeting malnutrition, promoting psychosocial development, parenting, and preschool educational interventions.

POLICY AND PROGRAMS

Policy and Training

Out of 16 LIC, National Policy for Child and Adolescent Mental Health existed only in 4, and only 3 countries reported that medicine was available free of cost to family and submitted data about CAMH to the Annual Health Survey.

As per the Child ATLAS Project, national-level epidemiology data were available from only 1 country; no country had child and adolescent mental health program or service outcomes data.[4,7] There was a lack of a continuum of care and universal barriers to access care for children and adolescents.[9] The acknowledgment of the UN Convention on the Rights of the Child, which is often seen as a corollary of child mental health policy, ratified by many low-resource countries far exceeds its use in policy or program development, and there is no evidence to suggest a correlation between the

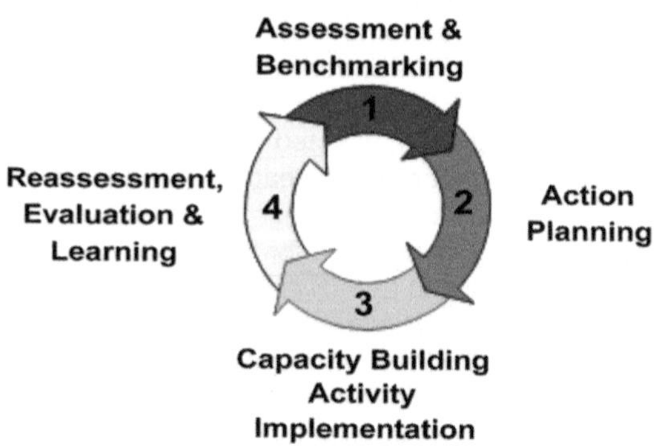

Fig. 5. Capacity building process.

convention ratification and the development of CAMH to support access to care and elimination of discrimination.[4,7]

The presence of informed, effective child mental health policy is critically important for the mental health of children. Policy guides the development of CAMH, advocacy for care, the assurance of access to care, and the remediation of gaps in care.[82] Policy is crucial to develop and sustain programs, provide oversight and accountability, and guides intersectorial collaboration. Often, policy, training, research, service provision, and human resources are interrelated (see **Fig. 2**).

Policy deficits are pervasive in high- and low-resource countries. In the WHO African Region, only 33.3% of countries had some form of child and adolescent mental health policy (not comprehensive) and only 6.3% of countries identified a child and adolescent mental health program.[83] Worldwide, only 7% of countries (14 of 191) had a clearly articulated, specific child and adolescent mental health policy.[83] Of the developing countries, Ghana, Lithuania, and South Africa have most substantially developed child and adolescent mental health policies.[4,7]

Nearly half a century has passed since the acknowledgment of the need for national-level policy in child and adolescent mental health (**Fig. 6**). Low-resource countries should be equally active and innovative in formulating national-level child and adolescent mental health specific policies and programs. Because adult or general mental health policy often lacks a developmental framework, it is not as reliant on support for intersectoral care. Therefore, there has to be a specific policy for child and adolescent mental health.

In some low-resource countries, mental health policies are available but are not comprehensive; for example, policies and programs are lacking or not well-coordinated, specifically related to children with autism spectrum disorders/mental health services related to the effects of war and/or natural disasters. Issues related to juvenile crime, child trafficking, domestic violence, for example, are often run by NGOs, but many times are not monitored by governments. These programs only address limited aspects of child and adolescent mental health with minimal or no coordination with the local health professionals. These resources can be better used for providing comprehensive child and adolescent psychiatric services. Efforts should be made to establish an integrated umbrella policy at a national level that is comprehensive, clear, objective, simple, culturally appropriate, and implementable.

Any effective policy should be able to prioritize needs, formulate effective strategies for addressing the needs, and provide evidence-based informed health care with a mandate to do no harm, for example, rational pediatric psychopharmacology, foster consensus, negotiate with the stakeholders, determine the specific areas of action,

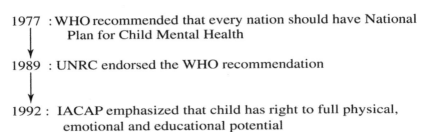

1977 : WHO recommended that every nation should have National Plan for Child Mental Health

↓

1989 : UNRC endorsed the WHO recommendation

↓

1992 : IACAP emphasized that child has right to full physical, emotional and educational potential

Fig. 6. Chronology of child mental health policies. IACAP, International Association for Computing and Philosophy; UNRC, United Nations Resident Coordinator; WHO, World Health Organization.

develop mechanism of governance structure, place mechanism(s) for periodic evaluation and monitoring, and include mechanisms of financing (without any negative competition between stakeholders or government bodies like ministry of education, health, and social welfare), including aspects of health insurance. Child and adolescent mental health funding is rarely identifiable in LAMIC and "out-of-pocket expenditure" is usually the practice in paying for services in 71.4% of the African countries. Each country's national budget must permanently allocate funds for such services. Other alternatives to generate funds should also be explored, such as social insurance and international grants. Ideally, every health sector at the district, state, or institutional level should have a rehabilitation unit where parents and families who have recovered or are recovering as a part of rehabilitation program can develop a coordinated revenue generating mechanisms (eg, by manufacturing candles) supervised by the institution or the government.

In developing countries, fewer than 40% of patients in the public sector and fewer than 30% in the private sector are being treated according to clinical practice guidelines (rational use of medicines: either prescribed, dispensed or sold). In this regard, the WHO recommends is the creation of special committees to monitor and improve the use of medications, training students in pharmacotherapy and prescription of drugs, removal of financial incentives for prescribers, establishment of criteria for ethical drug promotion, educating patients and parents, supervision of staff, and ensuring an adequate supply of drugs.[84]

Policy development depends on many factors.[85] As an example, in 2012, the "Nirbhay gang rape case" in new Delhi, the capital of India, created political instability in the country that forced the government to create the "Justice Verma Committee," which resulted in a rigorous reexamination of the existing laws for juvenile crime, and created a countrywide interest. This case has called for debate on minimum age of criminal responsibility (which is 18 years in India) for the juveniles. These heinous crimes committee by juveniles have raised the issue of lowering the age of criminal responsibility in India.

Creating skilled human resources is the most important challenge and cannot be met unless it is a part of the overarching health policy. This can be done via the "principle of task sharing" by capacity building among specialists, such as general adult psychiatrists, pediatricians, obstetricians, neurologists, general practitioners, clinical psychologists, and other mental health paraprofessionals (speech and language therapists, physiotherapists, occupational therapists, vocational educational specialists, medical and psychiatric social workers, mental health nurses, and general nurses). Supplemental training, direct training, short-term and long-term certificate courses, and regular courses can be offered to develop these professionals into a skilled child mental health workforce. Telepsychiatry and mobile health technology can be used to strengthen such training, wherever feasible. Creating subspecialty courses in child and adolescent psychiatry and developing a standard curriculum for the same has to be an important part of the planning and is an urgent need. Mandatory and exclusive child and adolescent psychiatry rotations should be required for 2 to 3 months for postgraduate psychiatry trainees and for 1 month for general medical graduates, at a national level, for all LAMIC countries. This can certainly bring a positive change in the long run.

Public–private partnerships and the introduction of health insurance/social insurance can be an important part of child and adolescent mental health policy.[86] Policymakers must acknowledge the impact of child and adolescent mental disorders on society[8] (see **Fig. 2**) and act accordingly without delay. Although evidence on the cost-effectiveness of promotive and preventive interventions are related to early childhood development programs, innovative approaches that are country and culture specific will help to overcome this challenge.[86] Finally, because there is no role model for policy, global leaders and leaders from LAMIC must collaborate and work together while formulating policy. We have gathered some examples from various low-resource countries.

SUGGESTED SYSTEMIC APPROACH FOR LOW-RESOURCE COUNTRIES

Two approaches are proposed at a systemic level (**Figs. 7** and **8**). First is a "bidirectional" or "top-down and bottom-up" approach, where the action plan must start from the top level (ie, policymakers, international and national professional associations and organizations), and simultaneously work must progress with available resources at the grassroots level.

The second approach includes a "horizontal extension and vertical depth," that is, continue to enhance awareness, extend services, facilitate multisectorial coordination, and encourage collaboration, while simultaneously increasing the depth of understanding and management of child and adolescent mental disorders. Conducting in-depth and prioritized, focused research with both clinical and public health emphases is important.

Advocacy, Policy, and Program Development in India

Child psychiatrists, like general psychiatrists, need to be the strongest advocates engaging with the government, politicians, and policymakers on the one hand, and with the public and communities on the other hand. In India, abysmally low indices on the state of health of children and human development have led the government to promulgate policies and programs in support of children at different age levels or stages of development. These include antenatal, prenatal, and perinatal care for the mother and child; immunization for infants; and midday meals for school children. The Government of India formulated an Integrated Child Development Scheme, a comprehensive package of "Child Welfare Scheme" with the objectives to improve the health and nutritional status of children 0 to 6 years of age; to lay the foundation for the psychological, physical, and social development of the child; to decrease the incidence of morbidity, mortality, malnutrition, and school dropout; and to educate the mother so as to enhance the capability of the mother to look after the health needs of her child. The National Policy for Children is aimed to protect children from neglect, cruelty, and exploitation by prohibiting the employment of children younger than 14 years in hazardous occupations; and establishing facilities for the special

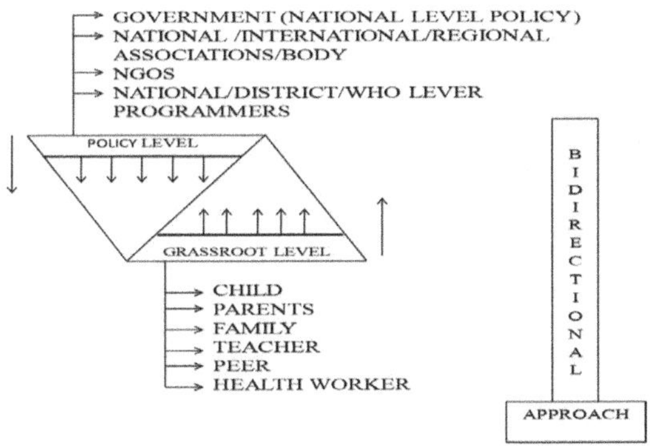

Fig. 7. "Bidirectional"/"top-down and bottom-up" approach. NGOs, nongovernmental organizations.

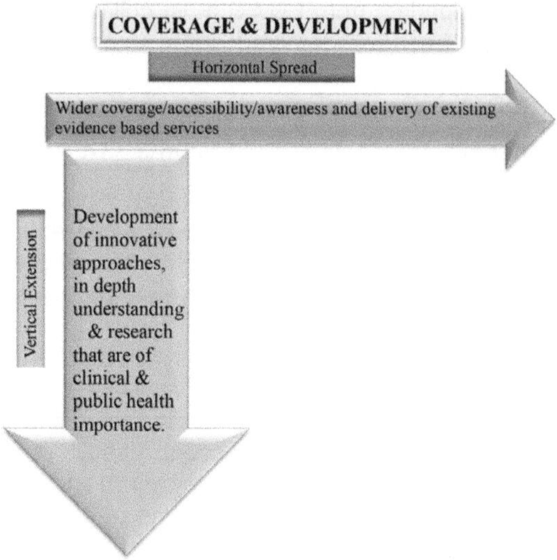
COVERAGE & DEVELOPMENT
Horizontal Spread
Wider coverage/accessibility/awareness and delivery of existing evidence based services
Vertical Extension
Development of innovative approaches, in depth understanding & research that are of clinical & public health importance.

Fig. 8. Horizontal extension and vertical depth approach.

treatment, education, utilization, and care of children who are physically handicapped, emotionally disturbed, or intellectually challenged. Further, amending existing laws so that, in all legal disputes between parents and/or institutions, the best interest of the child is always given paramount consideration. Child mental health issues are addressed indirectly through these development programs and, to that extent, remain embedded in the child development agenda generally. Child psychiatrists have come on to the stage only recently. A lot has been contributed by the active NGOs like "Action for Autism" in India, which has led to the formulation of the National Trust Act of 1999. The National Trust Act recognized autism, cerebral palsy, mental retardation, and multiple other conditions as disabilities. Making access to education a fundamental right has already pushed the demand for special education and counselors in schools in a significant way. Research in child psychiatry in India has provided evidence regarding the prevalence of mental health disorders in the country. Child mental health professionals have succeeded in bringing the issue of child mental health to the national agenda. The Ministry of Women and Child development, a program of the Government of India runs and advocates for a program namely "Beti Bachao Beti Padhao Scheme" (prevent female fetocide and educate the female child), Indira Gandhi Matritva Sahyog Yojana (IGMSY)" (improve the health and nutrition status of pregnant, lactating women and infants by providing cash incentive of Rs. 4000 in 3 installments between the second trimester and the time that the child turns 6 months of age). See also the "Rajiv Gandhi Scheme for Empowerment of Adolescent Girls (RGSEAG): Sabla" (available from: www.wcd.nic.in).

Professionals working in premier medical and psychiatric institutions who also serve on several decision making bodies/committees of the government through commitment and concerted effort have been able to focus national attention on several child mental health issues. Similarly, society in general and the media have contributed by bringing to public debate many issues, such as the right to education, inclusive education, and reforms for abandoned or neglected juveniles or the age of criminality for juveniles, which has propelled administrative and legal action on many fronts. India's commitment to many international treaties and conventions on child rights also contributed positively to enhancing services for them. A 3-year superspecialty course in Child and Adolescent Psychiatry at the National Institute of Mental Health and Neurosciences (NIMHANS) in Bangalore and at the Post-Graduate Institute of Medical Education and Research (PGIMER) in Chandigarh have been started in 2011 and 2014, respectively. The centers specialize in outpatient and inpatient programs along with community outreach services for children and adolescents with autism spectrum disorders, substance use or abuse, school mental health, and periodic training, workshops, and short courses. The development of a telepsychiatry software program for screening, diagnosing, formulating plan of management, and delivering psychosocial therapies in remote areas, with the support of primary care physician and community health workers, is a breakthrough in this regard.[42,45]

Advocacy, Policy, and Program Development in Other Low and Middle Income Countries

Lithuania

Lithuania has had child and adolescent psychiatry services being provided since 1990. It has 80 child and adolescent psychiatrists, 30 outpatient early intervention teams (for infants at risk of developmental disability like mental retardation, autism, cerebral palsy, and developmental problems), inpatient services, day care, crisis intervention services, and a mechanism to deliver a wide range of psychosocial interventions by a team of professionals stationed in the community.[7] Based on data from the World Bank from 2013, Lithuania has moved to the high-income category.

Vietnam

Vietnam has developed a model over 10 years, focusing on the development and delivery of CAMH services and research development.[87]

China

The 1-child policy in China has sparked concern among some people about the mental health consequences of growing up without siblings, and structural changes in entitlements have led some families to experience an escalation in stress that ultimately impacts the mental well-being of children.[82]

Brazil

New modalities of services have been developed in Brazil, demonstrating multidisciplinary collaboration within and between the health sector, educational system, and the judiciary. As mentioned, the role of the Equilibrium Project in Sao Paulo in developing a community-based and integrated approach for the street children is an important development.[48,81]

Turkey

The impact of public and government experience after 2 major earthquakes has created a window of opportunity and political will to transform national mental health policy in Turkey.[85]

Thailand

Thailand has a mobile child mental health service composed of a child psychiatrist, psychologist, and a social worker who provide new as well as follow-up care and child psychiatry consultations.[88]

Ethiopia

A 2-week child psychiatry course and a 4-week child psychiatry clinical internship (observe the behavior, assess the mental state of children with mental health problems, and trainers skill assessment at the end of posting) were implemented successfully during the first and the second years of the Masters of Science (MSC) program, respectively.[89]

Bangladesh

The following programs have been developed and implemented successfully: distance training for mothers of children with cerebral palsy to increase adaptive skills in children and mothers, and to underscore the importance of home-based care facilities[43]; benefit of a low-cost, school-based intervention, delivered by teachers in reducing conduct problems and increasing social skills at home and at school[34]; counselor-led school-based intervention in promoting resilience and mental health promotion in conflict affected Nepal and India.[90,91]

SUMMARY

Ninety percent of the world's children and adolescents live in low-income countries and about one-half of lifetime mental disorders begin before 14 years of age. The prevalence of child and adolescent mental disorders in low-resource countries is as great as in high-resource countries. Further, the resources are not only insufficient, but are also distributed inequitably and used inefficiently, with a treatment gap of more than 90%. Such challenges are exaggerated by already existing compromised health indices such as poverty, undernutrition, unemployment, an high occurrence of infectious diseases, and other social indices of low-resource countries. Specific, national-level child and adolescent mental health policy and standardized training are virtually nonexistent. Skilled human resources are extremely deficient. Many children and adolescents lack access to care. Effective mechanisms for systematic data gathering are absent. Qualitative and quantitative evidence on country- and culture-specific interventions have yet to be developed. There is the need to strengthen capacity building through supplemental training of the personnel who are working in an already existing and established health care program, by using innovative technologies like telepsychiatry and mobile health technology. Creating more employment opportunities in the field of child and adolescent mental health will attract more professionals to be engaged in providing care. The formulation of national-level and specific child and adolescent mental health policies, generating funds for collaborative and cross-cultural research, and creating more academic institutes providing superspecialty courses in child and adolescent psychiatry are urgently needed. Where there is a will, there is a way.

REFERENCES

1. Patel V, Kieling C, Maulik PK, et al. Improving access to care for children with mental disorders: a global perspective. Arch Dis Child 2013;98(5):323–7.
2. UNICEF. Statistics and monitoring. 2008. Available at: http://www.unicef.org/statistics. Accessed December 25, 2010.
3. Kessler RC, Berglund PM, Demler O, et al. Lifetime prevalence distributions of DSM-IV disorders in the national comorbidity study replication. Arch Gen Psychiatry 2005;62:593–602.
4. Belfer ML, Saxena S. WHO child Atlas project. Lancet 2006;367(9510):551–2.
5. WHO. World health report 2001—mental health: new understanding, new hope. Geneva (Switzerland): World Health Organization; 2001.
6. Verhulst FC. Epidemiology as a basis for the conception and planning of services. In: Remschmidt H, Belfer ML, Goodyer I, editors. Facilitating

pathways: care, treatment, and prevention in child and adolescent mental health. Berlin: Springer Verlag; 2004. p. 3–15.
7. World Health Organization (WHO). Atlas child and adolescent mental health resources—global concerns: implications for the future. 2005. Available at: http://www.who.int/mental_health/resources/Child_ado_atlas.pdf. Accessed October 3, 2005.
8. Morris J, Belfer M, Daniels A, et al. Treated prevalence of and mental health services received by children and adolescents in 42 low-and-middle-income countries. J Child Psychol Psychiatry 2011;52(12):1239–46.
9. Belfer ML. Child and adolescent mental disorders: the magnitude of the problem across the globe. J Child Psychol Psychiatry 2008;49(3):226–36.
10. Atlas: child, adolescent and maternal mental health resources in the Eastern Mediterranean Region. EMRO Technical Publication Series 2011;39:1–49.
11. Srinath S, Kandasamy P, Golhar TS. Epidemiology of child and adolescent mental health disorders in Asia. Curr Opin Psychiatry 2010;23(4):330–6.
12. Patel V, Kim YR. Contribution of low- and middle-income countries to research published in leading general psychiatry journals, 2002-2004. Br J Psychiatry 2007;190:77–8.
13. Patel V, Flisher AJ, Nikapota A, et al. Promoting child and adolescent mental health in low and middle income countries. J Child Psychol Psychiatry 2008; 49(3):313–34.
14. Kieling C, Baker-Henningham H, Belfer M, et al. Child and adolescent mental health worldwide: evidence for action. Lancet 2011;378(9801):1515–25.
15. Eaton J, McCay L, Semrau M, et al. Scale up of services for mental health in low-income and middle-income countries. Lancet 2011;378(9802):1592–603.
16. Kakuma R, Minas H, van Ginneken N, et al. Human resources for mental health care: current situation and strategies for action. Lancet 2011;378(9803):1654–63.
17. Klasen H, Crombag AC. What works where? A systematic review of child and adolescent mental health interventions for low and middle income countries. Soc Psychiatry Psychiatr Epidemiol 2013;48(4):595–611.
18. Leibson CL, Katusic SK, Barbaresi WJ, et al. Use and costs of medical care for children and adolescents with and without attention-deficit hyperactivity disorder. JAMA 2001;285:60–6.
19. Leslie DL, Rosenheck RA, Horwitz SM. Patterns of mental health utilization and costs among children in a privately insured population. Health Serv Res 2001;36:113–27.
20. Scott S, Knapp M, Henderson J, et al. Financial cost of social exclusion: followup study of anti-social children into adulthood. BMJ 2001;322:191–5.
21. Barbui C, Dua T, van Ommeren M, et al. Challenges in developing evidence-based recommendations using the GRADE approach: the case of mental, neurological, and substance use disorders. PLoS Med 2010;7(8).
22. Dua T, Barbui C, Clark N, et al. Evidence-based guidelines for mental, neurological, and substance use disorders in low- and middle-income countries: summary of WHO recommendations. PLoS Med 2011;8(11):e1001122.
23. World Health Organization. mhGAP intervention guide for mental, neurological, and substance use disorders in non-specialized settings. 2010. Available at: http://www.who.int/mental_health/evidence/mhGAP_intervention_guide/en/index.html. Accessed October 10, 2011.
24. Malhotra S, Chaturvedi SK. Patterns of childhood psychiatric disorders in India. Indian J Pediatr 1984;51(409):235–40.
25. Varma VK. Culture and the Indian personality. In: Varma VK, Kala AK, Gupta N, et al, editors. Culture, personality and mental illness: a perspective of traditional

Societies. New Delhi (India): Jaypee Brothers Medical Publishers (P)Ltd; 2009. p. 177–88.
26. Chen C-Y, Chieh-Yu L, Su W-C, et al. Factors associated with the diagnosis of neurodevelopmental disorders: a population-based longitudinal study. Pediatrics 2007;119:e435–43.
27. Malhotra S, Arun P, Kohli A. Applicability of Rutter-B scale on Indian population. Indian J Psychiatry 2000;42(1):66–72.
28. Polanczyk G, Silva de Lima M, Horta BL, et al. The worldwide prevalence of ADHD: a systematic review and metaregression analysis. Am J Psychiatry 2007;164:942–8.
29. Rescorla L, Achenbach TM, Almqvist F, et al. Epidemiological comparisons of problems and positive qualities reported by adolescents in 24 countries. J Consult Clin Psychol 2007;75:351–8.
30. Omigbodun OO. Psychosocial issues in a child and adolescent psychiatric clinic population in Nigeria. Soc Psychiatry Psychiatr Epidemiol 2004;39:667–72.
31. Panter-Bricka C, Eggermana M, Gonzalezb V, et al. Violence, suffering, and mental health in Afghanistan: a schoolbased survey. Lancet 2009;374: 807–16.
32. Prior M, Virasinghe S, Smart D. Behavioural problems in Sri Lankan schoolchildren, associations with socio-economic status, age, gender, academic progress, ethnicity and religion. Soc Psychiatry Psychiatrepidemiol 2005;40:654–62.
33. Hoven CW, Doan T, Musa GJ, et al. Worldwide child and adolescent mental health begins with awareness: a preliminary assessment in nine countries. Int Rev Psychiatry 2008;20(3):261–70.
34. Baker-Henningham H, Scott S, Jones K, et al. Reducing child conduct problems and promoting social skills in a middle-income country: cluster randomised controlled trial. Br J Psychiatry 2012;201:101–8.
35. Srinath S, Girimaji SC, Gururaj G, et al. Epidemiological study of child and adolescent psychiatric disorders in urban and rural areas of Bangalore, India. Indian J Med Res 2005;122:67–79.
36. Cho SM, Kim HS, Kim HJ, et al. Perceived need and use of child mental health services in Korea. Community Ment Health J 2009;45:56–61.
37. Shaffer D, Fisher PW, Lucas CP. Respondent-based interviews. In: Shaffer D, Lucas CP, Richters JE, editors. Diagnostic assessment in child and adolescent psychopathology. New York: Guilford Press; 1999. p. 3–33.
38. Burns BJ, Costello EJ, Angold A, et al. Children's mental health services use across services sectors. Health Aff 1995;14:147–59.
39. Khandelwal SK, Sharan P, Saxena S. Eating disorders: an Indian perspective. Int J Soc Psychiatry 1995;41:132–46.
40. Padhy SK, Khatana S, Sarkar S. Media and mental illness: relevance to India. J Postgrad Med 2014;60(2):163–70.
41. Becker AE. Body, self and society – the view from Fiji. Philadelphia: University of Pennsylvania Press; 1995.
42. Malhotra S, Chakrabarti S, Shah R. Telepsychiatry: promise, potential, and challenges. Indian J Psychiatry 2013;55(1):3–11.
43. McConachie H, Huq S, Munir S, et al. A randomized controlled trial of alternative modes of service provision to young children with cerebral palsy in Bangladesh. J Pediatr 2000;137(6):769–76.
44. Malhotra S, Chakrabarti S, Shah R, et al. Development of a novel diagnostic system for a telepsychiatric application: a pilot validation study. BMC Res Notes 2014;7:508.

45. Jensen PS, Goldman E, Offord D, et al. Overlooked and underserved: "action signs" for identifying children with unmet mental health needs. Pediatrics 2011; 128(5):970–9.
46. Wig NN, Murthy RS, Harding TW. A model for rural psychiatric services - Raipur Rani experience. Indian J Psychiatry 1981;23(4):275–90.
47. Malhotra S, Varma VK, Verma SK, et al. Childhood psychopathology measurement schedule: development and standardization. Indian J Psychiatry 1988; 30(4):325–31.
48. Scivoletto S, da Silva TF, Rosenheck RA. Child psychiatry takes to the streets: a developmental partnership between a university institute and children and adolescents from the streets of Sao Paulo, Brazil. Child Abuse Negl 2011;35(2):89–95.
49. Collins PY, Patel V, Joestl SS, et al. Grand challenges in global mental health. Nature 2011;475(7354):27–30.
50. Goodman A, Fleitlich-Bilyk B, Patel V, et al. Child, family, school and community risk factors for poor mental health in Brazilian school children. J Am Acad Child Adolesc Psychiatry 2007;46:448–56.
51. Datta SS, Premkumar TS, Chandy S, et al. Behaviour problems in children and adolescents with seizure disorder: associations and risk factors. Seizure 2005; 14:190–7.
52. Patel V, Goodman A. Researching protective and promotive factors in mental health. Int J Epidemiol 2007;36:703–7.
53. Graham P. The end of adolescence. Oxford (United Kingdom): Oxford University Press; 2004.
54. Fan F, Su L, Gill MK, et al. Emotional and behavioral problems of Chinese left-behind children: a preliminary study. Soc Psychiatry Psychiatrepidemiol 2010; 45(6):655–64.
55. Zakaria Z, Yaacob Bin MJ. Psychiatric morbidity among children and adolescents living in orphanages, Kota Bharu, Malaysia. Int Med J 2008;15:183–8.
56. Simşek Z, Erol N, Oztop D, et al. Epidemiology of emotional and behavioral problems in children and adolescents reared in orphanages: a national comparative study. Turk Psikiyatri Derg 2008;19:235–46 [in Turkish].
57. Frets-Van Buuren JJ, Letuma E, Daynes G. Observations on early school failure in Zulu children. S Afr Med J 1990;77(3):144–6.
58. Shenoy J, Kapur M, Kaliaperumal VG. Psychological disturbance among 5- to 8-year-old school children: a study from India. Soc Psychiatry Psychiatrepidemiol 1998;33(2):66–73.
59. Padhy SK, Goel S, Das SS, et al. Prevalence and patterns of learning disabilities in school going children in a northern city of India. Indian J Pediatr, in press.
60. Tramontina S, Martins S, Michalowski MB, et al. School dropout and conduct disorder in Brazilian elementary school students. Can J Psychiatry 2001;46:941–7.
61. Patel V, De Souza N. School drop-out: a public health approach. Natl Med J India 2000;13(6):316–8.
62. Patel V, Rahman A, Jacob KS, et al. Effect of maternal mental health on infant growth in low income countries: new evidence from South Asia [review]. BMJ 2004;328(7443):820–3.
63. Malhotra S. Challenges in providing mental health services for children and adolescents in India. In: Young JG, Ferrari P, editors. Designing mental health services and systems for children and adolescents: a shrewd investment. New York: Brunner/Mazel; 1998. p. 321–34.
64. Malhotra S, Kohli A, Arun P. Prevalence of psychiatric disorders in school children in Chandigarh, India. Indian J Med Res 2002;116:21–8.

65. Malhotra S, Varma VK, Verma SK. Temperament as determinant of phenomenology of childhood psychiatric disorders. Indian J Psychiatry 1986;28(4):263–76.
66. Hetherington EM, Bridges M, Insabella GM. What matters? what does not? Five perspectives on the association between marital transitions and children's adjustment. Am Psychol 1998;53(2):167–84.
67. Nikapota AD, Cox AD, Sylva K, Rai D. Development of culture appropriate child mental health services: perceptions and use of services. London: Department of Health; 1998.
68. Bhat PN, Arnold F, Gupta K, et al. Household population and housing characteristics. International Institute for Population sciences (IIPS) and Macro International. 2007. National Family Health Survey (NFHS-3), 2005–06: India: Volume I. Mumbai: IIPS.
69. Chadda RK, Deb KS. Indian family systems, collectivistic society and psychotherapy. Indian J Psychiatry 2013;55(Suppl 2):S299–309.
70. Loo SK, Rapport MD. Ethnic variations in children's problem behaviors: a cross-sectional, developmental study of Hawaii school children. J Child Psychol Psychiatry 1998;39(4):567–75.
71. Flisher AJ, Myer L, Mèrais A, et al. Prevalence and correlates of partner violence among South African adolescents. J Child Psychol Psychiatry 2007;48(6):619–27.
72. Leckman JF, Leventhal BL. Editorial: a global perspective on child and adolescent mental health. J Child Psychol Psychiatry 2008;49:221–5.
73. Patel V, Araya R, Chatterjee S, et al. Treatment and prevention of mental disorders in low-income and middle-income countries. Lancet 2007;370:991–1005.
74. Jordans MJD, Tol WA, Komproe IH, et al. Systematic review of evidence and treatment approaches: psychosocial and mental health care for children in war. Child Adolesc Ment Health 2009;14:2–14.
75. Flament MF, Nguyen H, Furino C, et al. Evidence-based primary prevention programmes for the promotion of mental health in children and adolescents: a systematic worldwide review. In: Remschmidt H, Nurcombe B, Belfer M, et al, editors. The mental health of adolescents. An area of global neglect. Chichester (England): Wiley; 2007. p. 65–136.
76. Available at: http://wcd.nic.in/icds.htm. Accessed July 2, 2015.
77. Available at: http://www.usaid.gov/indonesia/health. Accessed July 2, 2015.
78. Cuanto. 2003. "De Beneficiarios a Clientes: Aplicacion de la 'Libreta De Calificaciones' a Programas Sociales en Peru. Principales Resultados Relacionados al Programa No Escolarizado de Educacion Inicial (PRONOEI)." Lima. Available at: http://www.mef.gob.pe/contenidos/pol_econ/documentos/pronoei_final.pdf. Accessed March 7, 2015.
79. Available at: http://www.unicef.org/teachers/resources/child.htm. Accessed July 2, 2015.
80. Bernal R, Fernández C. Subsidized childcare and child development in Colombia: effects of Hogares Comunitarios de Bienestar as a function of timing and length of exposure. Soc Sci Med 2013;97:241–9.
81. Kieling C, Belfer M. Opportunity and challenge: the situation of child and adolescent mental health in Brazil. Rev Bras Psiquiatr 2012;4:241–4.
82. Belfer ML. Critical review of world policies for mental healthcare for children and adolescents. Curr Opin Psychiatry 2007;20(4):349–52.
83. Shatkin JP, Belfer ML. The global absence of a child and adolescent mental health policy. Child Adolesc Ment Health 2004;9:104–8.
84. Rational use of medicines, focusing on child mental health. vol. 375. Available at: www.thelancet.com. Accessed June 12, 2010.

85. Munir K, Tuncay E, Tunaligil V, et al. A window of opportunity for the transformation of national mental health policy in Turkey following two major earthquakes. Harv Rev Psychiatry 2004;12:238–51.
86. Zechmeister I, Kilian R, McDaid D, MHEEN Group. Is it worth investing in mental health promotion and prevention of mental illness? A systematic review of the evidence from economic evaluations. BMC Public Health 2008;8:20.
87. Weiss B, Ngo VK, Dang HM, et al. A model for sustainable development of child mental health infrastructure in the LMIC World: Vietnam as a case example. Int Perspect Psychol 2012;1(1):63–77.
88. Remschmidt H, Belfer ML, Goodyer I, editors. Facilitating pathways: care, treatment and prevention in child and adolescent mental health. Berlin: Springer; 2004.
89. Tesfaye M, Abera M, Gruber-Frank C, et al. The development of a model of training in child psychiatry for non-physician clinicians in Ethiopia. Child Adolesc Psychiatry Ment Health 2014;8(1):6.
90. Jordans MJ, Komproe IH, Tol WA, et al. Evaluation of a classroom-based psychosocial intervention in conflict-affected Nepal: a cluster randomized controlled trial. J Child Psychol Psychiatry 2010;51(7):818–26.
91. Rajaraman D, Travasso S, Chatterjee A, et al. The acceptability, feasibility and impact of a lay health counsellor delivered health promoting schools programme in India: a case study evaluation. BMC Health Serv Res 2012;12:127.

The Global Implications of Bullying and Other Forms of Maltreatment, in the Context of Migratory Trends and Psychiatric Resources

Jorge C. Srabstein, MD

KEYWORDS

- Bullying • Maltreatment • Global public health • Migration • Psychiatric resources

KEY POINTS

- Bullying is a multifaceted form of maltreatment, associated with other forms of victimization. It is prevalent across social settings, along the lifespan, and around the world.
- It is necessary to promote international awareness about the serious health and safety risks associated with bullying and other forms of victimization.
- The relevance of higher prevalence of bullying and other forms of maltreatment in certain parts of the world not only has significant public health bearing on those nations affected by them but also worldwide, because migrants carry with them the effects of victimization.
- Psychiatrists practicing in countries with a considerable migrant population should not only advocate for the mental health needs of migrants but also for the development of immigration policies that call for the clinical detection of prior victimization, not for the purpose of deterring the migratory process but, on the contrary, to ensure the provision of adequate health services and follow-up.

INTRODUCTION

There are a growing number of published studies showing a wide range of health problems affecting young people who participate in bullying incidents, as victims, perpetrators, or bystanders.[1–11] This situation demands a concerted effort of health professionals, and especially child and adolescent psychiatrists, in detecting and preventing bullying-related morbidity and mortality.[12–14] In this context clinicians may be faced with the emergent understanding of the multiple aspects of the notion of bullying

---

Conflict of interest: The author has no conflict of interest.
Department of Psychiatry, Children's National Medical Center, Montgomery County Outpatient Regional Center, 9850 Key West Avenue, Rockville, MD 20850, USA
E-mail address: jsrabste@cnmc.org

Child Adolesc Psychiatric Clin N Am 24 (2015) 799–810
http://dx.doi.org/10.1016/j.chc.2015.06.008 **childpsych.theclinics.com**
1056-4993/15/$ – see front matter

as a form of harm, which can be associated with other types of maltreatment,[15,16] taking place across different social settings[17–22] and around the world.[23]

According to Olweus'[24] initial definition, bullying is a multifaceted type of abuse characterized by the exposure of a student to intentional and repeated physical and or emotional maltreatment by 1 or more students. Furthermore, an imbalance of power is another requisite in Olweus'[25] pivotal research concept of bullying, because he stated that "it is not bullying when two students of about the same strength quarrel or fight."

Child and adolescent psychiatrists facing the need to identify the occurrence of a bullying incident may be challenged by the clinical constraints of determining whether the event meets the research requirements of intentionality, recurrence, and imbalance of power.

It may be difficult, in a clinical setting, to ascertain whether an incident of bullying has been committed deliberately. Furthermore, regardless of intentionality, a victim may still be hurt. Clinical limitations may also be encountered in determining whether there is an imbalance of dominance between the perpetrator and the victim. Again, both of them may be hurting each other, regardless of balance of power, as in the case of physical fights. Hence, a physical fight can be medically understood as mutual physical bullying, aggression, or mistreatment, in which all participants, regardless of balance of power, are simultaneously victims and perpetrators, at significant risk of being injured.[10] In addition, the need for bullying to be repetitive and over time, as specified in its original research concept, may be incongruent with the toxic effects of this form of abuse, because 1 episode may be enough to cause harm.[26]

In the process of evolving globalization it is relevant to emphasize that what is understood as bullying varies according to various cultures.[27] In some languages, words such as bullismo (Italian), mobbing (Swedish), ibbulijar (Maltese), and zorbalik (Turkish) can be literally translated into English as bullying. Other languages use terms for bullying such as kunyanyaswa (Swahili), dręczenia (Polish), and intimidare (Romanian), which respectively can be translated as abuse, harassment, and intimidation.

The notion of bullying, as a multifaceted type of maltreatment, encompasses the concepts of harassment, intimidation, abuse, aggression, violence, neglect, rejection, and exclusion. It can also be associated with many other forms of maltreatment, including assault, homicide, extortion, vandalism, human trafficking, ethnic conflict, rape, physical punishment, kidnapping, terrorism, and war.

The significant link of bullying with a wide array of health problems has been reported in different countries. These studies show a significant association between this form of maltreatment and alcohol consumption, posttraumatic stress disorder, psychosis, poor subjective health, headaches, stomach aches, dizziness, sleeping difficulties, irritability, suicidal risk, injuries, and depression.[28–34]

It has been estimated that almost 10% of adolescent students in the United States experience a cluster of physical and emotional symptoms linked to their participation in bullying incidents both as perpetrators and/or victims.[3] These students were 8.14 times more likely to hurt themselves on purpose and 4.20 times more likely to hurt others purposely compared with their peers who were not involved in bullying and who did not have a cluster of physical and emotional symptoms.[3]

There is a growing awareness that bullying can co-occur in the school milieu, at home among siblings, in dating relations, on cyberspace, in correctional facilities, and at the workplace.[17–22] Exposure to multiple forms of victimization has been documented to be common.[35] Thirty percent of US children and adolescents had been exposed to more than 1 type of victimization, and 10% experienced 11 or more different forms of victimization in their lifetime.[35]

A significant number of reports,[23,36–47] based on data from the World Health Organization (WHO) Global School-based Student Health Survey (GSHS)[48] and/or the Health Behavior in School-aged Children (HBSC) survey,[49] have documented the global prevalence of bullying, extending from the lowest (7%) in Tajikistan to the highest (70%) in Zimbabwe.[23] On average, one-third of adolescent students in 66 countries and territories around the world were bullied at school at least once in the previous 1 to 2 months.[23]

From a global perspective bullying is a broad term that encompasses many forms of maltreatment, such as intimidation, physical fights, verbal and nonverbal aggressive acts, and even mortality as in homicide. It is also important to examine the significance of bullying in this context to global migratory trends and the ready access to and availability of psychiatric resources.

GLOBAL PREVALENCE OF BULLYING

The HBSC and the GSHS include questions about bullying, which is defined by both surveys as an unpleasant thing being said or done to a student, being teased a lot in an unpleasant way, or being left out of things on purpose. Both surveys exclude from the concept of bullying a physical fight between 2 students of the same strength or power.

An examination of the HBSC and GSHS data from 121 countries or territories, over a period of 12 years (2001–2013), showed that an average of 28.5% of adolescents, aged 13 to 15 years, reported being bullied once, twice, or more frequently in the previous 1 to 2 months. The broad global distribution of adolescent bullying prevalence extends from a low 4% in Sweden and Finland to a maximum of 75% in Samoa, among the nations with the highest prevalence (ie, greater than the 95th percentile) (**Table 1**).

WORLDWIDE FREQUENCY OF ADOLESCENT PHYSICAL FIGHTS

Physical fights are significantly linked to bullying[10] and also, as previously discussed, they can be medically regarded as a type of mutual maltreatment, regardless of the balance of power between the parties and/or mutual agreement to be engaged in such an act. Reviewing the same HBSC and GSHS data set from 2001 to 2013 revealed that an average of 19% of adolescents aged 13 to 15 years were involved in at least 3 physical fights in the previous year worldwide. The frequency distribution of this form of reciprocal abuse extends from a minimum of 7% in Greenland to an upper limit of 71% in Tuvalu (see **Table 1**).

Physical Assault

According to the GSHS data in 66 countries and territories, an average of 38% of students, aged 13 to 15 years reported having been physically attacked once or more in the previous year. The lowest prevalence (10%) was documented in Kiribati and the highest frequency was reported in Samoa (see **Table 1**).

HOMICIDES

Homicides have been reported to be associated with incidents of bullying,[50] and they should be regarded as a type of maltreatment.[51] A review of the WHO database estimates show that, in 2012, there was a wide range in the prevalence of homicide rates per country, from a low of 0.2 per 100,000 population (Luxembourg) to the highest frequency, in Honduras, of 104 per 100,000 population[52] (see **Table 1**; **Table 2**).

Table 1
Countries and territories with highest prevalence[a] of bullying and/or other types of maltreatment

Countries	Bullying (%)	Physical Fights (%)	Physical Assaults (%)	Homicide[b]	Mortality Caused by Interpersonal Violence[c]
Zambia	63	—	—	—	—
Solomon Islands	67	53	—	—	—
Vanuatu	67	—	—	—	—
Egypt	69	—	—	—	—
Samoa	75	49	72	—	—
Zambia	—	53	—	—	—
Ghana	—	55	55	—	—
Botswana	—	56	—	—	—
Yemen	—	57	—	—	—
Djibouti	—	60	58	—	—
Tuvalu	—	71	—	—	—
Malawi	—	—	63	—	—
South Africa	—	—	—	35.7 per 100,000	—
Lesotho	—	—	—	37.5 per 100,000	—
Guatemala	—	—	—	39.9 per 100,000	—
Colombia	—	—	—	43.9 per 100,000	8.4 per 100,000
El Salvador	—	—	—	43.9 per 100,000	—

[a] 95th percentile.
[b] Rates per 100,000 population.
[c] Rates per 100,000 population aged 15 to 29 years.

MORTALITY CAUSED BY INTERPERSONAL VIOLENCE

Interpersonal violence has been defined as violent behavior or aggression between family members, intimate partners, acquaintances, and/or strangers that is not intended to further the aims of any formally defined group or cause.[53] This category includes child and elder abuse, intimate partner violence, sexual assault or rape, youth violence, aggression during property crimes, and violence in institutional settings.

A review of the WHO mortality data by cause in 173 countries, during 2012,[54] indicates that an average of 1.22 per 100,000 individuals, aged 15 to 29 years, died of interpersonal violence. Thirty percent of the countries reported a mortality of 0 per 100,000. Brazil is the highest among 9 countries with the highest rates of mortality (95th percentile) caused by interpersonal violence among youth (see **Tables 1** and **2**).

MORTALITY CAUSED BY COLLECTIVE VIOLENCE AND LEGAL INTERVENTION

Collective violence has been defined as "the instrumental use of violence by people who identify themselves as members of a group – whether this group is transitory or has a more permanent identity – against another group or set of individuals, in order to achieve political, economic or social objectives."[55] The notion of collective violence includes wars, terrorism, and other political conflicts, genocide, torture, repression, kidnappings and disappearance of individuals, gang warfare, and banditry.[55]

Table 2
Countries and territories with highest prevalence[a] of other types of maltreatment

Countries	Homicide[b]	Mortality Caused by Interpersonal Violence[c]	Mortality Caused by Collective Violence and Legal Intervention[c]
Belize	44.7 per 100,000	—	—
Jamaica	45.1 per 100,000	—	—
Venezuela	57.6 per 100,000	8.4 per 100,000	—
Honduras	103.9 per 100,000	—	—
Ethiopia	—	5.8 per 100,000	—
United States	—	7.4 per 100,000	—
Congo (Kinshasa)	—	10.3 per 100,000	—
Mexico	—	13.1 per 100,000	—
Nigeria	—	15.1 per 100,000	—
India	—	22.6 per 100,000	—
Brazil	—	34.0 per 100,000	—
Pakistan	—	—	2.9 per 100,000
Iraq	—	—	4.5 per 100,000
Afghanistan	—	—	7.0 per 100,000
Syria	—	—	27.1 per 100,000

[a] 95th percentile.
[b] Rates per 100,000 population.
[c] Rates per 100,000 population age 15 to 29.

The WHO's statistics on mortality caused by collective violence[54] are combined with rates of prevalence of deaths caused by legal intervention, or deaths caused by "injuries inflicted by the police or other law-enforcing agents, including military on duty, in the course of arresting or attempting to arrest lawbreakers, suppressing disturbances, maintaining order, and other legal action."[56] The highest 2012 WHO mortalities caused by collective violence and legal intervention, among persons 15 to 29 years old, were documented in Pakistan, Iraq, Afghanistan, and Syria, with a range of prevalence from 2.9 per 100,000 to 27.1 per 100,000 (see **Table 2**).

MIGRATION PATTERNS AND AVAILABILITY OF PSYCHIATRIC RESOURCES

According to the latest available United Nations' data on international migration,[57] as of 2013, there were an estimated 231.5 million foreign-born people residing in all countries of the world. From this data,[57] it can be calculated that approximately 27% of these migrants (63.34 million people) originated in one of the 32 countries with the highest prevalence (greater than 95th percentile) of bullying and other forms of maltreatment (see **Tables 1** and **2**).

Among the 10 countries with the largest migratory influx, there is a high percentage of migrant populations from countries with the highest prevalence of bullying and other forms of maltreatment or victimization: United Arab Emirates (61.56%), Saudi Arabia (55.90%), and the United States (47.09%) (**Table 3**). The largest migratory destinations for people from states with the highest frequency of one or more types of maltreatment are frequently nations other than those with the world's largest migratory influx (**Table 4**). In this context, there is a considerable migratory flow between Afghanistan and Iran, Iraq and Syria, Syria and Lebanon, and Colombia and Venezuela.

Table 3
Percentage of migrant stock from countries with high prevalence of types of maltreatment, among countries with highest migrant stock,* and the availability of psychiatric resources

Countries with Highest Migrant Stock	Migrant Stock* From Countries with High Prevalence of Types of Maltreatment (%)
United States	47.09
Russia	0.17
Germany	5.9
Saudi Arabia	55.9
United Arab Emirates	61.56
United Kingdom	30.14
France	4.94
Canada	21.92
Australia	11.28
Spain	14.83

Countries with available psychiatry resources (1.1 psychiatrist per 100,000 or more) are bolded. Those with limited psychiatric resources (<1.1 psychiatrist per 100,000) are not bolded.

* Migrant stock is the number of foreign-born or foreign citizens in 1 country. When data on place of birth are available, they are generally given precedence.

Table 4
Main migratory destination for countries with highest frequency of bullying and other forms of maltreatment, and availability of psychiatric resources

Country of Origin	Main Migratory Destination	Migrant Stock (%)[a]	Country of Origin	Main Migratory Destination	Migrant Stock (%)[a]
Afghanistan	**Iran**	86.00	Malawi	Zimbabwe	27.25
Belize	**United States**	0.11	**Mexico**	**United States**	28.28
Botswana	South Africa	2.00	Nigeria	United States	0.55
Colombia	**Venezuela**	70.77	Samoa	**New Zealand**	5.76
Congo (Kinshasa)	Congo (Brazzaville)	61.72	Solomon Islands	**New Zealand**	0.03
Djibouti	**France**	0.08	South Africa	**United Kingdom**	2.73
Egypt	**Saudi Arabia**	14.33	Syria	**Lebanon**	2.5
El Salvador	**United States**	2.99	Tuvalu	**New Zealand**	0.14
Ethiopia	**United States**	0.39	**United States**	**Mexico**	76.91
Ghana	Nigeria	14.3	Vanuatu	New Caledonia	7.68
Guatemala	**United States**	2.00	**Venezuela**	**United States**	0.47
Honduras	**United States**	1.20	Yemen	**Saudi Arabia**	5.08
India	United Arab Emirates	36.44	Zambia	South Africa	2.69
Iraq	Syria	54.00	—	—	—
Jamaica	**United States**	0.75	—	—	—
Lesotho	South Africa	12.95	—	—	—

Countries with available psychiatry resources (≥1.1 psychiatrist per 100,000) are bolded. Those with limited psychiatric resources (<1.1 psychiatrist per 100,000) are not bolded.

[a] Percentage of foreign-born or foreign citizens in 1 country of migratory destination who originated in a country with high prevalence of bullying and other forms of maltreatment.

Psychiatric Resources

In order to establish the availability of psychiatric resources at the countries with the highest rates of bullying and other types of victimization and their points of migratory destination, we examined the WHO database on rates of psychiatrists per 100,000 of population per country.[58] We chose the median, which is a rate of 1.1 psychiatrists per 100,000, as the point above or below which available psychiatric resources versus restricted psychiatric resources could be established.

Seventy-six percent of countries with the highest prevalence of bullying and/or other types of maltreatment have very restricted or unavailable psychiatric resources and only 30% of their main migratory destination countries have availability of resources (see **Table 4**).

IMPLICATIONS OF GLOBAL HIGH PREVALENCE OF BULLYING AND OTHER FORMS OF MALTREATMENT

The relevance of higher prevalence of bullying and other forms maltreatment in certain parts of the world has not only significant public health bearing on those nations affected by them but also worldwide, because migrants carry with them the effects of victimization.

It is important to highlight the significant risk for victimization in migrant communities,[59–64] which may compound the effects of poly victimization that may have been witnessed and/or experienced in the countries of origin and/or during, sometimes very hazardous, migrant journeys.

Given the significant public health responsibility of child and adolescent psychiatrists to prevent, detect, and treat the wide array of morbidity related to bullying and other forms of maltreatment, there first needs to be a focus on the urgent problem of a world in which 50% of the population lives in countries where there is less than 1 psychiatrist to serve 200,000 people.[58] This global public health crisis seriously affects those countries with high prevalence of different forms of maltreatment or victimization as well as many of those countries that are primary destinations for their migratory inflows. It is imperative that all health professionals be trained in the prevention, detection, and treatment of health problems related to all forms of maltreatment or victimization. In the context of evolving globalization the use of Tele Psychiatry and Tele Education in addition to sound public policies by legislators and local governments regarding these issues is warranted.

In those countries with available psychiatric resources and significant migrant populations it is incumbent on the mental health professionals there to be aware of the serious public risks that potentially can affect migrant communities, not only because of ongoing maltreatment but, above all, because of a significant high risk of previous multiple exposures to victimization. This requirement may result in the need to detect and treat clinical cases, manifested by a wide array of symptoms, including insomnia, nightmares, multiple physical symptoms, anxiety, marked mood instability, flashbacks, dissociation, inattention, impulsivity, aggression, substance abuse, and psychosis.[11]

Even if psychiatric resources are available in a host country, challenges persist, such as concerns about possible limitations to access to health care by migrants, depending on their legal immigration status and/or the health policies of the host country. Furthermore, there may be constraints in the understanding of the use of mental health resources depending on cultural differences and religious practices.

Psychiatrists practicing in countries with a considerable migrant populations should not only advocate for the mental health needs of migrants but also for the development of immigration policies that call for the clinical detection of prior victimization, not for the purpose of deterring the migratory process but, on the contrary, to ensure the provision of adequate health services and follow-up.

There is a need for a more comprehensive global public health research, involving child and adolescent psychiatrists, in ascertaining the psychobiosocial factors resulting in higher rates of prevalence of bullying and other forms of maltreatment, around the world.

This article focuses on the highest prevalence of maltreatment, operationally defined as greater than the 95th percentile. Ongoing efforts should identify a broader group of nations with high victimization prevalence by including, at least, all countries with rates in the 90th percentile and by widening the scope of maltreatment to include other facets like sexual assault as well as mind and human trafficking.

Furthermore there is a need to promote international awareness about the serious health and safety risks associated with bullying and other forms of maltreatment, across social settings and along the life span. To fulfill this objective there is an emergent international nonprofit project known as the Global Health Initiative for the Prevention of Bullying (GHIPB).[65] Its main initial goal is to reach out to medical educators around the world to foster the inclusion in medical curriculums of knowledge about the nature, ecology, epidemiology, detection, and prevention of morbidity related to bullying and other forms of maltreatment. Above all, GHIPB intends to promote a worldwide recognition that the morbidity and mortality linked to bullying constitute a major international public health concern.[13] Its prevention will require the joint effort of health practitioners, educational and industry organizations, families, and communities.[12] Such prevention strategies could help nations preserve safe and healthy living and the learning and working conditions of their inhabitants, while reducing expenditure on bullying-related disease and the immeasurable and overwhelming cost related to premature loss of life.[13]

REFERENCES

1. Litwiller BJ, Brausch AM. Cyber bullying and physical bullying in adolescent suicide: the role of violent behavior and substance use. J Youth Adolesc 2013; 42(5):675–84.
2. Farrant B, Utter J, Ameratunga S, et al. Prevalence of severe obesity among New Zealand adolescents and associations with health risk behaviors and emotional well-being. J Pediatr 2013;163(1):143–9.
3. Srabstein J, Piazza T. Is there a syndrome of bullying? Int J Adolesc Med Health 2011;24(1):91–6.
4. Arslan S, Hallett V, Akkas E, et al. Bullying and victimization among Turkish children and adolescents: examining prevalence and associated health symptoms. Eur J Pediatr 2012;171(10):1549–57.
5. Luk JW, Wang J, Simons-Morton BG. The co-occurrence of substance use and bullying behaviors among U.S. adolescents: understanding demographic characteristics and social influences. J Adolesc 2012;35(5):1351–60.
6. Idsoe T, Dyregrov A, Idsoe EC. Bullying and PTSD symptoms. J Abnorm Child Psychol 2012;40(6):901–11.
7. Nixon CL, Linkie CA, Coleman PK, et al. Peer relational victimization and somatic complaints during adolescence. J Adolesc Health 2011;49(3):294–9.
8. Klomek AB, Kleinman M, Altschuler E, et al. High school bullying as a risk for later depression and suicidality. Suicide Life Threat Behav 2011;41(5):501–16.
9. Rivers I. Morbidity among bystanders of bullying behavior at school: concepts, concerns, and clinical/research issues. Int J Adolesc Med Health 2011;24(1):11–6.

10. Srabstein J, Piazza T. Public health, safety and educational risks associated with bullying behaviors in American adolescents. Int J Adolesc Med Health 2008; 20(2):223–33.
11. Srabstein JC, McCarter RJ, Shao C, et al. Morbidities associated with bullying behaviors in adolescents. School based study of American adolescents. Int J Adolesc Med Health 2006;18(4):587–96.
12. Srabstein J, Joshi P, Due P, et al. Prevention of public health risks linked to bullying: a need for a whole community approach. Int J Adolesc Med Health 2008;20(2):185–99.
13. Srabstein JC, Leventhal BL. Prevention of bullying-related morbidity and mortality: a call for public health policies. Bull World Health Organ 2010;88(6):403.
14. Srabstein J. Working towards a detection of bullying related morbidity. Int J Adolesc Med Health 2012;24(1):77–82.
15. Turner HA, Finkelhor D, Shattuck A, et al. Recent victimization exposure and suicidal ideation in adolescents. Arch Pediatr Adolesc Med 2012;166(12): 1149–54.
16. Finkelhor D, Ormrod RK, Turner HA. Polyvictimization and trauma in a national longitudinal cohort. Dev Psychopathol 2007;19(1):149–66.
17. Espelage DL, De La Rue L. School bullying: its nature and ecology. Int J Adolesc Med Health 2011;24(1):3–10.
18. Wolke D, Skew AJ. Bullying among siblings. Int J Adolesc Med Health 2012; 24(1):17–25.
19. Ellis WE, Wolfe DA. Bullying predicts reported dating violence and observed qualities in adolescent dating relationships. J Interpers Violence 2014. [Epub ahead of print].
20. Hinduja S, Patchin J. Bullying beyond the schoolyard. Preventing and responding to cyberbullying. 1st edition. Thousand Oaks (CA): Corwin Press; 2009.
21. Ireland JL. Understanding bullying among younger prisoners: recent research and introducing the multifactor model of bullying in secure settings. Int J Adolesc Med Health 2011;24(1):63–8.
22. Einarsen S, Hoel H, Zapf D, et al. Bullying and emotional abuse in the workplace. International perspectives in research and practice. London: Taylor & Francis; 2003.
23. Due P, Holstein BE, Soc MS. Bullying victimization among 13 to 15-year-old school children: results from two comparative studies in 66 countries and regions. Int J Adolesc Med Health 2008;20(2):209–21.
24. Olweus D. Bullying at school: what we know and what we can do? Oxford (United Kingdom): Blackwell; 1993. p. 9.
25. Olweus D. Norway. In: Catalano R, Junger-Tas J, editors. The nature of school bullying: a cross national perspective. London: Routledge; 1999. p. 30.
26. Srabstein JC. The prevention of bullying: a whole school and community model. In: Shute RH, Slee PT, Murray Harvey R, et al, editors. Mental health and well-being: educational perspectives. Adelaide (Australia): Shannon Research Press; 2011. p. 299.
27. Smith PK, Monks CP. Concepts of bullying: developmental and cultural aspects. Int J Adolesc Med Health 2008;20(2):101–12.
28. Pierobon M, Barak M, Hazrati S, et al. Alcohol consumption and violence among Argentine adolescents. J Pediatr (Rio J) 2013;89(1):100–7.
29. Kelleher I, Harley M, Lynch F, et al. Associations between childhood trauma, bullying and psychotic symptoms among a school-based adolescent sample. Br J Psychiatry 2008;193(5):378–82.

30. Gobina I, Zaborskis A, Pudule I, et al. Bullying and subjective health among adolescents at schools in Latvia and Lithuania. Int J Public Health 2008;53(5):272–6.
31. Due P, Holstein BE, Lynch J, et al. Bullying and symptoms among school-aged children: international comparative cross sectional study in 28 countries. Eur J Public Health 2005;15(2):128–32.
32. Kim YS, Koh YJ, Leventhal B. School bullying and suicidal risk in Korean middle school students. Pediatrics 2005;115(2):357–63.
33. Laflamme L, Engström K, Möller J, et al. Bullying in the school environment: an injury risk factor? Acta Psychiatr Scand Suppl 2002;412:20–5.
34. Saluja G, Iachan R, Scheidt PC, et al. Prevalence of and risk factors for depressive symptoms among young adolescents. Arch Pediatr Adolesc Med 2004;158(8):760–5.
35. Turner HA, Finkelhor D, Ormrod R. Poly-victimization in a national sample of children and youth. Am J Prev Med 2010;38(3):323–30.
36. Siziya S, Rudatsikira E, Muula AS. Victimization from bullying among school-attending adolescents in grades 7 to 10 in Zambia. J Inj Violence Res 2012;4(1):30–5.
37. Granero R, Poni ES, Escobar-Poni BC, et al. Trends of violence among 7th, 8th and 9th grade students in the state of Lara, Venezuela: The Global School Health Survey 2004 and 2008. Arch Public Health 2011;69(1):7.
38. Siziya S, Muula AS, Rudatsikira E. Prevalence and correlates of truancy among adolescents in Swaziland: findings from the Global School-Based Health Survey. Child Adolesc Psychiatry Ment Health 2007;1(1):15.
39. Rudatsikira E, Siziya S, Kazembe LN, et al. Prevalence and associated factors of physical fighting among school-going adolescents in Namibia. Ann Gen Psychiatry 2007;6:18.
40. Erginoz E, Alikasifoglu M, Ercan O, et al. The role of parental, school, and peer factors in adolescent bullying involvement: results from the Turkish HBSC 2005/2006 Study. Asia Pac J Public Health 2015;27(2):NP1591–603.
41. Vieno A, Gini G, Santinello M. Different forms of bullying and their association to smoking and drinking behavior in Italian adolescents. J Sch Health 2011;81(7):393–9.
42. Harel-Fisch Y, Walsh SD, Fogel-Grinvald H, et al. Negative school perceptions and involvement in school bullying: a universal relationship across 40 countries. J Adolesc 2011;34(4):639–52.
43. Wang J, Iannotti RJ, Nansel TR. School bullying among adolescents in the United States: physical, verbal, relational, and cyber. J Adolesc Health 2009;45(4):368–75.
44. Craig W, Harel-Fisch Y, Fogel-Grinvald H, et al. A cross-national profile of bullying and victimization among adolescents in 40 countries. Int J Public Health 2009;54(Suppl 2):216–24.
45. Molcho M, Craig W, Due P, et al. Cross-national time trends in bullying behaviour 1994-2006: findings from Europe and North America. Int J Public Health 2009;54(Suppl 2):225–34.
46. Alikasifoglu M, Erginoz E, Ercan O, et al. Bullying behaviours and psychosocial health: results from a cross-sectional survey among high school students in Istanbul, Turkey. Eur J Pediatr 2007;166(12):1253–60.
47. Schnohr C, Niclasen BV. Bullying among Greenlandic schoolchildren: development since 1994 and relations to health and health behaviour. Int J Circumpolar Health 2006;65(4):305–12.

48. World Health Organization, Chronic Diseases and Health Promotion, Global School-based Student Health Survey (GSHS). Available at: http://www.who.int/chp/gshs/en/. Accessed October 14, 2014.
49. World Health Organization, Health Behaviour in School-aged Children (HBSC). Available at: http://www.euro.who.int/en/health-topics/Life-stages/child-and-adolescent-health/adolescent-health/health-behaviour-in-school-aged-children-hbsc2.-who-collaborative-cross-national-study-of-children-aged-1115. Accessed October 16, 2014.
50. Srabstein J. Deaths linked to bullying and hazing. Int J Adolesc Med Health 2008;20(2):235–9.
51. Srabstein JC. News reports of bullying-related fatal and nonfatal injuries in the Americas. Rev Panam Salud Publica 2013;33(5):378–82.
52. World Health Organization, Global Health Observatory Data Repository, homicide estimates by country. 2012. Available at: http://apps.who.int/gho/data/node.main.VIOLENCEHOMICIDE?lang=en. Accessed January 1, 2015.
53. Waters H, Hyder A, Rajkotia Y, et al. The economic dimensions of interpersonal violence. Geneva (Switzerland): Department of Injuries and Violence Prevention, World Health Organization; 2004. p. 2. Available at: http://whqlibdoc.who.int/publications/2004/9241591609.pdf. Accessed January 1, 2015.
54. World Health Organization, Health Statistics and Information Systems, cause specific mortality, disease and injury country mortality estimates, 2000–2012, WHO member states, 2012, all persons, age 15-29, injuries, intentional injuries. Available at: http://www.who.int/healthinfo/global_burden_disease/estimates/en/index1.html. Accessed January 1, 2015.
55. Chapter 8. In: Krug EG, et al, editors. World report on violence and health. Geneva (Switzerland): World Health Organization; 2002. Available at: http://whqlibdoc.who.int/publications/2002/9241545615_eng.pdf?ua=1. Accessed January 1, 2015.
56. ICD version 2015, legal interventions and operations of war, Y35. Available at: http://apps.who.int/classifications/icd10/browse/2015/en#/Y35-Y36. Accessed January 1, 2015.
57. United Nations. Department of Economic and Social Affairs (2013). Trends in international migrant stock: migrants by destination and origin (United Nations database, POP/DB/MIG/Stock/Rev.2013). Table 10 Total migrant stock at mid-year by major area, region country or area of destination. 2013. Available at: http://www.un.org/en/development/desa/population/migration/data/estimates2/estimatesorigin.shtml. Accessed January 1, 2015.
58. World Health Organization. Global Health Observatory, mental health human resources per 100,000 population. 2011. Available at: http://www.who.int/gho/mental_health/human_resources/psychiatrists_nurses/en/Accessed January 1, 2015.
59. Hjern A, Rajmil L, Bergström M, et al. Migrant density and well-being–a national school survey of 15-year-olds in Sweden. Eur J Public Health 2013;23(5):823–8.
60. von Grünigen R, Perren S, Nägele C, et al. Immigrant children's peer acceptance and victimization in kindergarten: the role of local language competence. Br J Dev Psychol 2010;28(Pt 3):679–97.
61. Vieno A, Santinello M, Lenzi M, et al. Health status in immigrants and native early adolescents in Italy. J Community Health 2009;34(3):181–7.
62. Zadnik E, Sabina C, Cuevas CA. Violence against Latinas: the effects of undocumented status on rates of victimization and help-seeking. J Interpers Violence 2014. [Epub ahead of print].

63. Sela-Shayovitz R. The role of ethnicity and context: intimate femicide rates among social groups in Israeli society. Violence Against Women 2010;16(12):1424–36.
64. Strohmeier D, Kärnä A, Salmivalli C. Intrapersonal and interpersonal risk factors for peer victimization in immigrant youth in Finland. Dev Psychol 2011;47(1):248–58.
65. Global Health Initiative for the Prevention of Bullying (GHIPB). Available at: http://www.ghipb.org/. Accessed January 1, 2015.

Psychological Impact of Nuclear Disasters in Children and Adolescents

Finza Latif, MD[a,*], Jessica Yeatermeyer, MD, MSc[a], Zachary D. Horne, MD[b], Sushil Beriwal, MD[b]

KEYWORDS

- Nuclear disasters • Psychological impact • Children • Safety systems
- Radiation exposure

KEY POINTS

- There is a need for further investigation not only of the impact of nuclear disasters on children but also of whether the consequences are a direct result of the disaster, radiation exposure, or the psychosocial disruptions resulting from the disaster.
- Nuclear disasters are unique because they are man-made and represent a failure of the safety systems put in place to contain exceedingly dangerous radioactive materials.
- An increase in anxiety is observed in children immediately following the disaster and dissipates with time.
- Cancer and birth deformities can result from direct radiation exposure and may result in secondary psychological distress, although specific literature regarding this outcome is not available.
- There is a high level of resilience in children and it is important to treat parental anxiety in order to reduce the psychological impact on children.

INTRODUCTION

Nuclear disasters are devastating in several ways. The psychological impact is 2-fold: the direct impact of the disaster and the impact of any physical changes as a result of exposure to nuclear radiation. Overall, the rates of psychological impairment range from 25% to 75%, depending on the population under study, the timing of the assessments, the perceived or actual magnitude of the exposure, and the degree of direct involvement with the accident.

Conflicts of interest: None.
[a] Children's National Health System, George Washington University School of Medicine, 111 North Michigan Avenue, P1 W, Washington, DC 20010, USA; [b] University of Pittsburgh Cancer Institute, 5150 Centre Avenue, Pittsburgh, PA 15232, USA
* Corresponding author. Children's National Health System, George Washington University School of Medicine, 111 North Michigan Avenue, P1 W 10043, Washington, DC 20010.
E-mail address: flatif@childrensnational.org

Child Adolesc Psychiatric Clin N Am 24 (2015) 811–822
http://dx.doi.org/10.1016/j.chc.2015.06.009 childpsych.theclinics.com
1056-4993/15/$ – see front matter

Abbreviations

CBCL	Child Behavior Checklist
EEG	Electroencephalogram
GAD	Generalized anxiety disorder
ICD-10	International Classification of Diseases and Related Health Problems, Tenth Revision
IQ	Intelligence quotient
MDD	Major depressive disorder
OR	Odds ratio
PCL-S	PTSD Checklist Stressor Specific
PTSD	Posttraumatic stress disorder
RR	Risk ratio
TMI	Three Mile Island

Three of the largest nuclear disasters, namely Three Mile Island (TMI) Chernobyl, and Fukushima, which occurred in the United States, western Soviet Union (now Ukraine), and Japan respectively, are described in this article. This article reviews the literature and assesses the psychological and physical impact of these disasters on children and adolescents.

REVIEW OF MAJOR NUCLEAR DISASTERS

TMI is the worst nuclear disaster reported in the United States and it occurred at a plant near Harrisburg, Pennsylvania, in March 1978. Cooling water contaminated with radiation drained into adjoining buildings because of valve failure. Although no deaths were reported, approximately 140,000 people evacuated the area. There is controversy over whether there have been increased rates of cancer and infant mortality secondary to the incident. The Pennsylvania Department of Health maintained a registry of more than 30,000 people who lived within 5 miles of TMI at the time of the accident for 18 years. The state's registry was discontinued in 1997, without any evidence of unusual health trends in the area.[1] The Chernobyl incident is one of the worst disasters in history and occurred in April 1986 in Ukraine. An explosion and fire at the nuclear power plant released large quantities of radioactive particles into the atmosphere, which spread over much of the western Soviet Union and Europe. Thirty-one people died and more than 500,000 workers were exposed. Around 150,000 residents had to be evacuated and relocated.

The Fukushima Daiichi nuclear disaster occurred in March 2011 in Japan. An 8.9-magnitude earthquake led to a tsunami that then caused a series of equipment failures, nuclear meltdowns, and release of radioactive materials at the Fukushima nuclear power plant in eastern Japan. Around 300,000 people evacuated the area, thousands of people died because of the earthquake and tsunami, and thousands more died secondary to the evacuation conditions, such as living in temporary housing and hospital closures. In addition, contaminated water spread to the surrounding environment and the food supply. It was the largest nuclear disaster since the Chernobyl disaster.

Nuclear disasters are unique because there is an acute incident and then a period of contamination that can have a prolonged so-called silent exposure period, leading to both physical and psychological health effects. As Carl Sagan[2] describes in *Billions and Billions*, the exponential nature of the decay prolongs the remnant effects of radiation significantly. However, most studies do not quantify the radiation dosage of the exposure when assessing the psychological impact.

That these disasters have a psychological impact is undisputed. After TMI, the President's Commission concluded that the biggest public health problem was mental health. Twenty years after Chernobyl, the Chernobyl Forum similarly concluded that the biggest public health problem from Chernobyl was mental health (United Nations 2006).

Various factors determine the nature of psychological response to disaster. The disaster and subsequent disruption in day-to-day life, including loss of homes, evacuation, and adjustment to a new environment, are just a few of the contributing stressors. Another contributor to psychological distress is the fear of the physical impact of radiation (eg, cancer or limb deformities). There are several reports of individuals exposed to radiation being stigmatized and ostracized within their communities. The physical effects of radiation are discussed in more detail later in the article.

Furthermore, the individual's perception of the disaster is as important as the disaster itself in determining the psychological response. This factor is especially important in nuclear disasters because often the magnitude of the disaster and exposure rates are unknown and further misinformation from authorities, confusing media reports, and rumors may lead to the perception of a higher-than-actual risk. Surveys done 10 and 11 years after TMI and Chernobyl, respectively, with mothers of young children showed that those who thought that their health was affected by the disaster were 3 times more likely to report their current health as fair to poor compared with those who did not.[3] Similarly, adolescents who grew up in the vicinity of the Chernobyl accident had higher negative risk perception than their nonevacuee peers; less negative than their mothers' risk perception and only modestly associated with their actual mental health.[4] The response can also vary based on degree of controllability, predictability, the relative success of attempts to minimize injury to oneself or others, and whether there was actual loss.[5] Nuclear disasters occur because of failure of controls put in place and are unpredictable and therefore highly distressing.

In children, developmental stage and cognitive functioning also affect their response. Broadly, posttraumatic responses can be categorized into 3 realms: affective, behavioral, and cognitive. Very young children (0–2 years) may respond with increased separation anxiety, regression, or feeding problems. Slightly older children (2–7 years) may respond with insomnia, nightmares, increased worries, noise sensitivity, or irritability. Primary school children (7–11-year-olds) may show more anger, aggression, and acting out similar to adolescents (12–18-year-olds). The older age group may also display more fear or specific worries, sadness, cognitive distortions (eg, self-blame or generalization of negative view) and risk-taking behavior, like substance abuse or self-injury.

In addition, and perhaps most importantly, the response of parents plays an important role in how children respond to stress. Parents' conduct and coping is are predictors that can considerably alleviate or strengthen unfavorable effects of stress or trauma on a child's development. Therefore, the impact of nuclear disasters on adults is an important factor for children because there is a significant correlation between maternal psychosocial adaptation and the manifestation of stress in children. Long-term follow-up studies in adults affected by nuclear disasters have shown increased rates of self-reported medical problems, depression, anxiety and posttraumatic symptoms, and perception of decreased emotional well-being. For example, the lifetime prevalence of depression in women in the Ukraine is 20.8%,[6] whereas the lifetime prevalence of depression in women 11 years after Chernobyl was 46.7%. Mothers of young children have been identified as one of the 2 highest-risk population groups in nuclear disasters; the other being nuclear power plant workers, and this is a consistent finding despite the varied cultural context in which these nuclear disasters have occurred.

PHYSICAL EFFECTS OF RADIATION

Acute Effects

The immediate concern after exposure to radiation is the acute radiation syndrome, which consists of 3 phases and manifests over a period of minutes to days. The prodromal phase can present with nausea; vomiting; fatigue; and, in the most severe cases, diarrhea, fever, and hypotension. The latent phase follows, in which no symptoms are experienced. The duration of this phase is inversely proportional to the dosage of radiation exposure. This phase is followed by the acute illness phase. The timing and severity of this phase also depends on radiation dosage. In its most severe form it presents with microvasculature breakdown in the central nervous system. This breakdown can result in severe nausea, vomiting, altered mental status, poor coordination, acute respiratory distress, seizures, and ultimately coma and death.

Another physical manifestation is the gastrointestinal syndrome. The symptoms start 3 to 10 days following exposure. As the name implies, symptoms include nausea and vomiting, and severe (and often fatal) diarrhea. These symptoms occur because of destruction of intestinal crypt stem cells by radiation and reduce the ability of the gut to repopulate sloughed gastrointestinal villi. Even low doses can result in the hematopoietic syndrome, which consists of a depopulation of hematopoietic stem cells over a period of months. This syndrome results in increased rates of infection, bleeding, and anemia. In this situation, infections are the chief cause of death and can be mitigated with supportive care.[7,8]

Long-term Effects

In the regions surrounding nuclear reactor accidents and in people who survive the acute radiation syndromes, the primary concern is an increase in rates of cancer, especially in children exposed in utero and in vivo.

THYROID CANCER

A few studies have found a 30% to 50% increase in the incidence of thyroid cancer in the counties surrounding TMI.[9,10] Several studies have found a strong dose-response relationship between radiation dose to the thyroid received in childhood after Chernobyl and thyroid cancer risk.[1,11,12] The International Agency for Research suggests that the accident may have caused 1000 cases of thyroid cancer and 4000 cases of other malignancy throughout Europe. Further, the model predicts that by 2065 an additional 16,000 and 25,000 cases of thyroid and other malignancies, respectively, could be expected.[13] Data regarding increased rates of thyroid cancer after Fukushima are limited. A cross-sectional study of 1222 adolescents failed to correlate thyroid cancer diagnoses with radiation exposure.[14]

OTHER CANCERS

A significant correlation between proximity to TMI and cancer incidence was noted (odds ratio [OR] = 1.4), with lymphoma having the strongest association (OR = 1.9). However, after adjusting for confounding risk factors such as cigarette smoking, results were reduced to borderline significance.[15]

A cohort mortality study with a large cohort (30,135) noted a trend toward an increased risk of breast cancer, lymphoma, and leukemia based on estimated dose exposure in the TMI area.[1]

A second cohort study from University of Pittsburgh of 21,494 subjects older than 18 years in the region around TMI showed no increase in incidence of all malignancy, after adjusting for socioeconomic factors.[11] Higher doses of radiation exposure were related to increased rates of bronchogenic carcinoma in both men and women (risk ratio [RR] = 1.45) as well as leukemia in men (RR = 1.15).[11]

In-utero Exposure and Birth Defects

Aside from the risk of developing a malignancy as a result of in-utero radiation exposure, there is also a substantial risk of birth defects. Following Chernobyl, 96,438 births were evaluated and showed higher rates of neural tube defects, microcephaly, and microphthalmia compared with the European average.[12] Increased rates of trisomy-21 have also been correlated to in-utero radiation exposure in several European countries in the years following Chernobyl.[16,17]

PSYCHOLOGICAL EFFECTS OF RADIATION

In examining children's psychological well-being after the nuclear disasters at TMI, Chernobyl, and the Fukushima Daiichi power plant, we reviewed data and outcomes from 3 review articles (2 focusing on Chernobyl alone and 1 assessing studies of all 3 disasters) and 15 original articles (10 regarding Chernobyl, 2 regarding TMI, and 3 regarding Fukushima). Taken together, these studies evaluated more than 4800 children who ranged in age from in utero to adolescence at the time of exposure and who were assessed at various intervals ranging from 2 months to 18 years after exposure. The studies reviewed used both subjective and objective measures to assess for psychological effects in children and their parents, and many of the studies include age-matched, gender-matched, and culturally matched control groups for comparison. The mental health data from these studies can be conceptualized into 4 primary categories: depressive and anxiety disorders (5 studies),[3,4,6,18–20] posttraumatic stress symptoms (2 studies),[20,21] behavior-related symptoms and attention/hyperactivity (2 studies),[3,6] and cognitive and intellectual functioning (7 studies).[6,22–29]

Depressive and Anxiety Disorders

Children exposed to radiation in the 3 identified disaster zones were evaluated for depression, anxiety, and somatization disorders using subjective measures predominantly, including self-rating scales such as the Children's Manifest Anxiety Scale, the Depression Self-rating Scale, the Youth Self-report, the Children's Depression Inventory, and several independent/nonstandardized scales particular to individual studies.[4,6,18–20] To assess parents' perceptions of internalizing and externalizing behavior problems in their children, several study groups used the Child Behavior Checklist (CBCL), the Child Symptom Inventory, the Behavior Screening Questionnaire, the Strengths and Difficulties Questionnaire, and other independently developed scales.[6,19,20,26,30,31] In order to explore possible relationships between parental distress and child symptoms, several groups also used self-rating scales to assess parent symptoms of depression, anxiety, and somatization, including the Symptom Checklist-90, the Schedule for Affective Disorders and Schizophrenia–Lifetime, the State-Trait Anxiety Inventory, and other nonstandardized questionnaires developed specifically for particular studies.[21,23,26,30] A specific scale was used in 1 study to detect so-called Chernobyl stress in mothers; an "8-item scale focused on the health effects of the Chernobyl disaster on mother and child, effects on future generations, and worries about eating or drinking contaminated food or milk."[6] Some studies also included more objective measures to assess mood and anxiety conditions in children and their parents, conducting psychiatric diagnostic interviews following International Classification of Diseases and Related Health Problems, Tenth Revision (ICD-10) or Diagnostic and Statistical Manual of Mental Disorders, Fourth Edition, criteria.[4,22–24,26]

Eleven years after the disaster at Chernobyl, Bromet and colleagues[6] used self-reports to evaluate 300 children who had been evacuated from the area in utero or as infants, and evacuees reported no difference in their general well-being compared with classmates in their new city. However, the mothers of these evacuees reported more somatic symptoms in their children than the control group, and there was a positive correlation between the mothers' levels of Chernobyl stress (explained earlier) and the somatic complaints they registered for their children. When this same cohort was evaluated at age 19 years (N = 265), using self-rating scales and formal psychiatric interviews, there was no difference detected in rates of major depressive disorder (MDD) and generalized anxiety disorder (GAD) compared with controls (7.2% in evacuees, 10.0% in relocation-area classmate controls, and 11.3% in population controls). Despite these diagnostic data, the teenagers rated their overall health as less satisfactory than the controls and they reported more health problems and medical diagnoses, even though there were no significant differences between the groups on physical examinations and laboratory tests. The investigators concluded that, although adolescents were more likely than their peers to believe that Chernobyl had negatively affected their health, and their parents were more likely to identify health concerns in their children if their Chernobyl stress was high, these perceptions of risk were not associated with diagnoses of MDD and GAD. Adjusting for known risk factors, the greatest identifiable predictors for MDD and GAD in this study were self-esteem, peer support, life events (unrelated to the nuclear accident), and female gender; risk factors that are not unique to the disaster literature.[4] Personal estimations of the risk associated with Chernobyl therefore affected symptom reports but not diagnosable conditions in both parents and children in these studies.

Similarly no difference was found in a 2010 study from Norway, evaluating adolescents living in a radiation far-field fallout region of the Chernobyl disaster. The study administered youth self-reports to teenagers who were in utero at the time of the disaster and child behavior checklists to their mothers. Problems reported by adolescents were low (mean total score of 31.5, which is lower than known regional numbers, although the specific control number is not reported in the study). Problems reported by mothers were even lower than those reported by the adolescents (mean total score on CBCL of 11.8, which is lower than numbers found in 3 other studies of norms for the region: 14.2, 15.4, and 13.6). The investigators posit that the lapse in time between the event and the study may account, in part, for the discrepancy between their data and those of other studies, because worries tend to dissipate with time. The investigators also suggest that the lack of an evacuation in Norway may have affected the emotional consequences after the disaster, because evacuation has been an identified confounder in studies from the highly affected regions. In addition, the investigators question whether certain protective factors in their study population (eg, higher socioeconomic status, readily available health care, and state-provided economic compensation for affected farmers) may account for the differences in their findings.[19]

Contrasting the aforementioned studies, a 1999 study by Kolominsky and colleagues[23] did find an increase in ICD-10 diagnosable emotional disorders in children exposed to the Chernobyl disaster. The study evaluated 250 children exposed versus unexposed in utero (respondents N = 138 and 122, respectively) at ages 6 to 7 years and 10 to 11 years using formal psychiatric interviews. There was a significant difference in rates of emotional disorders with onset specific to childhood (20.3% vs 7.4% at ages 6 to 7 years and 18.1% vs 7.4% at ages 10–11 years). The most frequently cited explanation of emotional disorders for both age groups was phobic anxiety (12.3% vs 5.6%; $P \leq .05$). For children in the exposed group, the most identifiable specific feature of phobic anxiety disorder was the fear of radiation and, considering the other stressors of the disaster (disruption of life by evacuation, resettling, and the economic and cultural hardships accompanying those activities), the investigators posit that these unfavorable social-psychological and social-cultural factors played a significant role in the cause of the emotional disturbances detected in children.

As in the studies from Chernobyl, the correlation between stress, emotional disturbance, and somatic complaints was also seen in a 1981 study by Dohrenwend and colleagues,[18] evaluating seventh, ninth, and eleventh graders living in the region of the TMI disaster (N = 632). The research group measured anxiety and somatic symptoms 2 months after the accident, asking respondents to rate their experiences during and immediately after the event, and at the 2-month mark. On a scale rating distress from 1 to 5, the average score during and immediately after the event was 3.25. Scores were higher for children who had a preschool-aged sibling living in the home (3.75 vs 3.12) and for children whose families left the area in response to the disaster (3.5 vs 3). The investigators related these differences to the level of worry within the family unit, positing that families with small children and families who deemed the disaster serious enough to leave the area registered higher levels of stress in general. For all groups, there was a sharp decrease in the level of stress 2 months after the event (with an average score of 2), but the decrease in score was not as great for children whose families left the area (2.25 vs 1.75), again suggesting that risk perception affects symptom reporting. In addition, somatic complaints were measured and although overall ratings were low, subjects reporting higher psychological distress also reported higher rates of somatic symptoms. Ultimately, the investigators concluded (1) that there was an immediate effect of psychological distress in the community, (2) that this effect dissipated over time, and (3) that respondents' perception of vulnerability influenced their symptoms. Note that there was no control group sampled in this study.[10] Another study measuring behavior problems of 3-year-olds who were infants at the time of the TMI accident indicated that 68% of exposed mothers expressed concern that their children's health would be affected because of their proximity to the disaster, but there was no significant difference in behavior problems of exposed and nonexposed children (rates of 13.2% in exposed boys and 9.2% in exposed girls compared with 11% in the general community).[9]

Data regarding children's internalizing behaviors after the more recent Fukushima plant disaster are not as developed as those for TMI and Chernobyl, and many of the available studies focus on the earthquake and tsunami without highlighting the nuclear plant effects specifically. Fujiwara and colleagues[31] showed that parental CBCL reports of children 5 to 7 years old who were preschoolers at the time of the earthquake (N = 178) rated higher internalizing problems (28%) than externalizing behaviors (21%) and that children who lost distant relatives or friends were more likely to show internalizing problems (47.6% vs 20.2%). Respondents were asked to rate the number of trauma events they endured in light of the tragedy (using the Trauma Events Screening Inventory) and most events reported were caused by the earthquake and its effects; however, 28% of respondents did list restrictions on their lifestyle caused by radiation as a trauma. The investigators write: "it remains unclear which [trauma] exposure is associated with which mental disorder or behavior problem". Regarding this question about the nuclear-specific effects of the Fukushima disaster, a 2014 review article by Bromet and colleagues[32] notes that preliminary data from several studies indicate that the emotional effects in that region are similar to those from Chernobyl and TMI in that cleanup workers and mothers of young children seem to be particularly at risk for developing mental health conditions.[33] Given the connection between maternal symptoms and child health noted earlier, similar effects may be expected to be seen in pediatric populations in the Fukushima region. Bromet[32] notes, "...having been exposed to multiple hazards, the health and mental health needs of the population affected by the triple disaster are inextricably intertwined."

Posttraumatic Stress Symptoms

Regarding posttraumatic stress disorder (PTSD), the nuclear disaster–specific data for children are scant. In 2011 and 2012, Yabe and colleagues[20] administered surveys by mail to more than 200,000 Japanese residents who lived in evacuation zones of the Fukushima disaster and assessed for affective and trauma-related disorders in children and adults, using PTSD Checklist Stressor Specific (PCL-S). However, the results for children and adults were reported jointly. For all respondents to the PCL-S (N = 60,704 in 2011 and 32,246 in 2012), 21.6% in 2011 and 18.3% in 2012 reported significant trauma symptoms and 25.0% reported social dysfunction secondary to trauma symptoms. The investigators concluded that there are "severe traumatic problems in adults from the evacuation zones," but they made no specific mention of PTSD in children. A study by Korol and colleagues[21] evaluated PTSD in Ohio children who were exposed to the inappropriate disposal of toxic waste in 1984. The Child PTSD Reaction Index was used to assess children directly and the Parent PTSD Reaction Index was used to measure how parents rated their children's trauma symptoms. Intrusion symptoms were rated highest by the children, but less than 7% of children overall rated high levels of PTSD. Parent psychological instability was the greatest predictor of child PTSD symptoms, a finding that is consistent with other data presented in this article suggesting that children's mental health after nuclear disaster is affected, if not predicted, by parental emotional well-being.[4,6,18,31,32] It is important also to note that the acuity of this incident was reportedly much lower than in the other nuclear disasters discussed in this article.[4,21]

BEHAVIOR AND ATTENTION/HYPERACTIVITY PROBLEMS

Bromet and colleagues[6] in their study 11 years after the Chernobyl disaster detected no difference in teacher-rated Conners scores (5.93 ± 6.00 vs 5.38 ± 5.42; $P>.05$) between the subject and control classmates. A similar study conducted 12 to 15 years after the disaster administered Conners Rating Scales–Revised to 1629 children and their mothers. The children's self-rated scores were within the normal range (T score <50) and there were no differences in scores based on degree of radiation exposure or whether the children were in utero or toddlers at the time of the disaster. Mothers' scores were higher than their children's ($P<.001$) on each of the Conners subscales, but most were still within normal or borderline (T score, 56–60) range. Mothers whose subjective perceptions were that their children's health was poor rated their children higher on the Conners scale, and mothers who were pregnant at the time of the incident rated their children significantly higher than mothers who were not pregnant. However, these discrepancies did not correlate positively with the objective measures of children's cognitive ability (using the Raven Standard Progressive Matrices Test, 1996 edition).[29] These findings are in line with those reported earlier for anxiety and somatic symptoms, suggesting that maternal stress levels and symptoms significantly affect child mental health reports, regardless of whether objective findings are in support or to the contrary.

COGNITIVE AND INTELLECTUAL FUNCTIONING

Cognitive functioning, particularly that of children who were exposed to nuclear radiation while in utero, has been the subject of many studies. To assess cognition, objective measures have been used by several different study groups, including electroencephalogram (EEG) studies, classroom grades, and academic test results, and neuropsychological testing in the form of the Wechsler Intelligence Scale for Children III, the Raven Standard Progressive Matrices Test (1996 edition), the Trail-making Test, the Wechsler Adult Intelligence Scale, the Hopkins Verbal Learning Test, the Visual Search and Attention Test, and the Benton Visual Retention Test.[6,22–24,26,27,29] Altogether, research groups using these measures evaluated 1094 children who were exposed to the Chernobyl disaster in utero or as toddlers, and the findings of these studies have been mixed. Litcher and colleagues[24] found no significant differences between exposed children and age-matched controls on any objective data measures (attention, memory, intelligence quotient [IQ], school grades) conducted when the children were 11 years old, or when the children were studied again at 19 years of age.[6,27] Two studies comparing 250 children exposed in utero with 250 controls, evaluated at ages 6 to 7 years and again at ages 10 to 12 years, detected lower mean full-scale IQ for the exposed versus the unexposed group (89.0 $\pm$ 9.6 vs 92.1 $\pm$ 8.7 in 6 to 7-year-olds $P \leq .01$; 93.7 $\pm$ 10.2 vs 96.1 $\pm$ 9.0 in 10–11-year-olds; $P \leq .05$), but found no dose-response difference in IQ levels based on the amount of radiation exposure.[22,23] The investigators attributed the discrepancies between exposed and unexposed children primarily to social-psychological and social-cultural factors, like parental education level, the stress of evacuation, and the breakdown of social contacts and difficulties with adapting to new surroundings after relocation.[23] Another study of 50 children exposed in utero versus 50 controls, assessed at ages 9 to 10 years, showed a significant difference in abnormal EEG patterns (74% vs 10%, respectively), and attributed this risk to radiation, showing a dose-response effect.[26] In sum, the existing studies of the quantifiable cognitive effects of nuclear disaster are discrepant at best and show a need for further inquiry.

LIMITATIONS OF EXISTING STUDIES

Several challenges exist in evaluating the effects of nuclear disaster on the mental health of children. Many studies note that it is difficult, if not impossible, to assess the amount of radiation to which each study participant was exposed, and how/where to draw geographic boundaries for exposed and unexposed regions.[4,6,18–20,22–24,29] Most studies that used control groups were able to find age-matched and gender-matched samples, but many of the studies noted that there were likely cultural differences between the 2 groups, particularly in studies involving evacuees who relocated to different regions or countries,[4,6,24,26,29] and 2 studies surveyed exposed groups but did not survey control groups.[18,19] Similarly, several studies noted that it was difficult to find region-specific norms for standardized tests, particularly with respect to neuropsychological testing, making it difficult to draw conclusions about unstudied baseline populations.[4,24,26] Also along those lines, several studies noted that interviewers in local sites were at times inexperienced in particular study methodology, especially in settings administering neuropsychological testing.[24,26,27] In addition, nearly all of the studies included in this article cite confounding socioeconomic and sociocultural factors of the regions examined, and the studies of the Fukushima disaster in particular note that the triple-disaster (ie, tsunami, earthquake, and nuclear meltdown) nature of the event makes it difficult to attribute findings to radiation exposure specifically.[20,31]

SUMMARY

In conclusion, the findings from longitudinal studies on mood and emotional well-being in nuclear disaster–exposed children suggest that somatic expressions of stress predominate. An increase in anxiety is observed in children immediately following the disaster and dissipates with time. In addition, perceptions of risk from the disasters significantly affect reports of depressive and anxiety symptoms in children but do not predict diagnoses. Anxiety about how bad the disaster will be for health, even for future generations, is a consistent outcome, although it is more significant in adults than in children. Most studies conclude that maternal perception of the impact of the disaster on their children is high. However, the rates of MDDs, GADs, PTSD, and attention-deficit/hyperactivity disorder are not higher in exposed children versus nonexposed children, when controlled for related disruptions in life (eg, evacuation, economic and social difficulties, parent education level). Such psychosocial disruptions may have a larger negative impact on the emotional well-being of children than the disaster and radiation exposure. However, cancer and birth deformities can result from direct radiation exposure, and may result in secondary psychological distress, although specific literature regarding this outcome is not available. Overall, these findings speak to a high level of resilience in children and the importance of treating parent anxiety in order to reduce the psychological impact on children.

REFERENCES

1. Talbott EO, Youk AO, McHugh-Pemu KP, et al. Long-term follow-up of the residents of the Three Mile Island accident area: 1979-1998. Environ Health Perspect 2003;111(3):341–8.
2. Sagan C. Billions and billions: thoughts on life and death at the brink of the millennium. New York: Penguin Random House Publishing Group; 1997. ISBN 0-679-41160-7.
3. Adams RE, Bromet EJ, Panina N, et al. Stress and well-being in mothers of young children 11 years after the Chornobyl nuclear power plant accident. Psychol Med 2002;32(1):143–56.
4. Bromet EJ, Guey LT, Taormina DP, et al. Growing up in the shadow of Chornobyl: adolescents' risk perceptions and mental health. Soc Psychiatry Psychiatr Epidemiol 2011;46(5):393–402.
5. Yehuda R. Post-traumatic stress disorder. N Engl J Med 2002;346(2):108–14.
6. Bromet EJ, Goldgaber D, Carlson G, et al. Children's well-being 11 years after the Chornobyl catastrophe. Arch Gen Psychiatry 2000;57:563–71.
7. Dörr H, Meineke V. Acute radiation syndrome caused by accidental radiation exposure - therapeutic principles. BMC Med 2011;9(1):126.
8. Christodouleas JP, Forrest RD, Ainsley CG. Short-term and long-term health risks of nuclear-power-plant accidents. N Engl J Med 2011;364:2334–41.
9. Levin RJ. Incidence of thyroid cancer in residents surrounding the Three Mile Island nuclear facility. Laryngoscope 2008;118(4):618–28.
10. Levin RJ, De Simone NF, Slotkin JF, et al. Incidence of thyroid cancer surrounding three mile Island nuclear facility: the 30-year follow-up. Laryngoscope 2013;123(8):2064–71.
11. Han YY1, Youk AO, Sasser H, et al. Cancer incidence among residents of the Three Mile Island accident area. Environ Res 2011;111(8):1230–5.

12. Wertelecki W. Malformations in a Chornobyl-impacted region. Pediatrics 2010; 125:e836–43.
13. Cardis E, Krewski D, Boniol M, et al. Estimates of the cancer burden in Europe from radioactive fallout from the Chernobyl accident. Int J Cancer 2006;119(6): 1224–35.
14. Watanobe H, Furutani T, Nihei M, et al. The thyroid status of children and adolescents in Fukushima Prefecture examined during 20-30 months after the Fukushima nuclear power plant disaster: a cross-sectional, observational study. PLoS One 2014;9(12):e113804.
15. Hatch MC, Wallenstein S, Beyea J, et al. Cancer rates after the Three Mile Island nuclear accident and proximity of residence to the plant. Am J Public Health 1991;81(6):719–24.
16. Sperling K, Neitzel H, Scherb H. Evidence for an increase in trisomy 21 (Down syndrome) in Europe after the Chernobyl reactor accident. Genet Epidemiol 2012;36(1):48–55.
17. Bromet EJ, Havenaar JM. Psychological and perceived health effects of the Chernobyl disaster: a 20-year review. Health Phys 2007;93(5):516–21.
18. Dohrenwend BP, Dohrenwend BS, Warheit GJ, et al. Stress in the community: a report to the president's commission on the accident at Three Mile Island. Ann N Y Acad Sci 1981;365:159–74.
19. Heiervang KS, Mednick S, Sundet K, et al. The psychological well-being of Norwegian adolescents exposed in utero to radiation from the Chernobyl accident. Dev Neuropsychol 2010;35(6):643–55.
20. Yabe H, Suzuki Y, Mashiko H, et al. Psychological distress after the Great East Japan Earthquake and Fukushima Daiichi Nuclear Power plant accident: results of a mental health and lifestyle survey through the Fukushima Health Management Survey in FY2011 and Fy2012. Fukushima J Med Sci 2014;60: 57–67.
21. Korol M, Green BL, Gleser GC. Children's responses to a nuclear waste disaster: PTSD symptoms and outcome prediction. J Am Acad Child Adolesc Psychiatry 1999;38(4):368–75.
22. Igumnov S, Drozdovitch V. The intellectual development, mental and behavioural disorders in children from Belarus exposed in utero following the Chernobyl accident. Eur Psychiatry 2000;15(4):244–53.
23. Kolominsky Y, Igumnov S, Drozdovitch V. The psychological development of children from Belarus exposed in the prenatal period to radiation from the Chernobyl atomic power plant. J Child Psychol Psychiatry 1999;40(2):299–305.
24. Litcher L, Bromet EJ, Carlson G, et al. School and neuropsychological performance of evacuated children in Kyiv 11 years after the Chornobyl disaster. J Child Psychol Psychiatry 2000;41(3):291–9.
25. Matsumoto J, Kunii Y, Wada A, et al. Mental disorders that exacerbated due to the Fukushima disaster, a complex radioactive contamination disaster. Psychiatry Clin Neurosci 2014;68(3):182–7.
26. Nyagu A, Loganovsky KN, Loganovskaja TK. Psychophysiologic aftereffects of prenatal irradiation. Int J Psychophysiol 1998;30(3):303–11.
27. Taormina DP, Rozenblatt S, Guey LT, et al. The Chernobyl accident and cognitive functioning: a follow-up study of infant evacuees at age 19 years. Psychol Med 2008;38(4):489–97.
28. World Health Organization. Health consequences of the Chernobyl accident. Results of the IPHECA pilot projects and related national programmes. Geneva (Switzerland): World Health Organization; 1995.

29. Bar Joseph N, Reisfeld D, Tirosh E, et al. Neurobehavioral and cognitive performances of children exposed to low-dose radiation in the Chernobyl accident. Am J Epidemiol 2004;160(5):453–9.
30. Cornely P, Bromet E. Prevalence of behavior problems in three-year-old children living near Three Mile Island: a comparative analysis. J Child Psychol Psychiat 1986;27(4):489–98.
31. Fujiwara T, Yagi J, Homma H, et al. Clinically significant behavior problems among young children 2 years after the Great East Japan Earthquake. PLoS One 2014;9(10):e109342.
32. Bromet EJ. Emotional consequences of nuclear power plant disasters. Health Phys 2014;106(2):206–10.
33. Bromet EL, Havenaar LM, Guey LT. A 25 year retrospective review of the psychological consequences of the Chernobyl accident. Clin Oncol (R Coll Radiol) 2011; 23(4):297–305.

Global Child and Adolescent Mental Health

A Culturally Informed Focus

Lisa M. Cullins, MD[a,*], Ayesha I. Mian, MD[b]

KEYWORDS

• Global • Mental health • Children • Culture • Collaboration

KEY POINTS

- There is a significant burden of mental illness in children and families across the globe.
- Despite heightened awareness of the significance of global mental health and its determinants on public health, there is an increased need for innovative interventions, research, resources, and efforts devoted to this area.
- It has been clearly established that culture is at the heart of this labor.
- In order to integrate culture into global mental health advocacy and solutions, a collaborative approach with flexibility in thinking and implementation must exist.

The Global Burden of Disease (GBD) was first published in 1996 by Murray and Lopez.[1,2] One of its key findings was that mental disorders were among the major causes of disability in high-income countries and low- and middle-income countries (LMICs). The investigators of the GBD study estimated that depression alone caused more disability than either nutritional problems or human immunodeficiency virus (HIV), which were then the prime foci of US health-related international programs.[1] At present, the World Health Organization (WHO) rates depression as the single greatest cause of disability worldwide, affecting at least 350 million people.[1] The 2010 GBD study showed that mental disorders account for 7.4% of the world's burden of health conditions in terms of disability-adjusted life years and nearly a quarter of all years lived with disability, more than cardiovascular diseases or cancer.[3] The global economic costs of mental disorders were estimated at $2.5 trillion in 2010 and are projected to reach $6 trillion by 2030.[3] Based on the above-mentioned findings, the WHO Action Plan recognized mental health as a global priority in May 2013. As a result of this pledged action, mental health is now discussed at the highest level policy forums devoted to global health and development. On the scientific side, after more

[a] 111 Michigan Avenue, NW, Washington, DC 20010, USA; [b] Department of Psychiatry, The Aga Khan University Hospital, Stadium Road, Karachi 74800, Pakistan
* Corresponding author.
E-mail address: LCullins@childrensnational.org

Child Adolesc Psychiatric Clin N Am 24 (2015) 823–830
http://dx.doi.org/10.1016/j.chc.2015.06.010 childpsych.theclinics.com
1056-4993/15/$ – see front matter

than a decade of sustained efforts to build knowledge, more innovations are evolving to successfully address the health and social needs of people with mental disorders.[3] Although mental illness is still striving for parity with all other medical illnesses, there is a global movement in the right direction.

Culture is defined as a shared dynamic system of values, beliefs, and lifestyles and evolves as needed to adapt to changing environmental conditions. Culture plays a clear role in its impact on the advancement of global mental health. If ignored and unaddressed, it acts as a barrier to change. On the other hand, if thoughtfully integrated, and if resources, engagement, and treatments are sensitized to cultural contexts, it can act as a powerful promoter of positive change, affecting the life trajectories of children and adolescents across the globe.

There is a steady stream of literature supporting the need for consideration of culture at every level of development—from needs assessment to implementation and sustainability, an individualized approach to the country, region, and village must ensue. The acceptability and use of mental health services are governed strongly by cultural attitudes, beliefs, and practices.[4]

CULTURE AND CULTURAL COMPETENCY

Culture is the integrated pattern of human behaviors including thoughts, communication, actions, customs, beliefs, values, and institutions of a racial, ethnic, religious, or social nature.[4] Cultural competence is a set of congruent behaviors, attitudes, and policies found in a system, agency, or professionals that enables them to work effectively in a context of cultural differences.[4] Although many traditional cultural values and beliefs are a source of strength and support for diverse children and families, some can act as barriers to mental health services. Stigma, belief systems as it pertains to symptoms and treatment, language, as well as resources are some of the most important elements to consider when addressing culture and global mental health.

Stigma can be a powerful barrier to timely access to treatment. In many cultures, mental illness has strong negative connotations, leading to the fear of double discrimination, preventing families from accessing services.[4] In some cultures, the stigma of mental illness extends far beyond the individual with the illness and to the family as a whole. For instance, in some cultures, it may be more difficult to marry if diagnosed with a mental disorder.[1] Stigma carries multiple layers of complexity. Children and adolescents in particular, in certain global areas plagued by violence, war, and illness (HIV/AIDS), may endure both the stigma of mental illness and the added stigma of having lost their family of origin to violence or HIV/AIDS, which ironically is more often the primary cause of their emotional distress and dysfunction.

Expressions of psychological or emotional distress differ across cultures. Idioms of distress are linguistic or somatic patterns of experiencing and expressing illness and/or general stress. Idioms of distress at times correlate with Westernized psychopathology but more often are unique psychological expressions of a given culture, which may actually be perceived as normative within that cultural context.[4] In some cultures, somatic manifestations of illness and/or symptoms are more prominent than others. More complex expressions of illness or distress are termed cultural syndromes.[4]

Language links connect us to our cultural roots. In health care, there is the physical examination that requires observations, touch, and medical instruments. But clinical examination would not be complete without the therapeutic engagement of the doctor/patient in which essential information is gleaned from the history taking and eliciting of pertinent signs and symptoms. Oral communication is essential in clinical assessments and treatment plans. In urban settings, there may be a predominance of one language, but most communities are multilingual. In mental illness, linguistic capability is imperative to examine and treat children and families. So often, there are extreme linguistic barriers to mental health treatment when interpreting resources are not available. Using the identified child (patient) as a language broker has been shown to do more harm than good. Language brokering, the common practice of having children act as interpreters between parents and medical professionals, should be avoided. High use of language brokering has been associated with higher levels of family stress, decrease in parenting effectiveness, poorer adjustment in academic functioning, higher Child Behavior Checklist internalizing scores, and substance use in adolescents.[4]

GLOBAL CHALLENGES IN CHILD AND ADOLESCENT MENTAL HEALTH

When thinking about global mental health and providing early intervention and treatment to children, adolescents, and families across the world, a collaborative approach is essential. Many gains have been made in looking at promising global practices as it pertains to the provision of mental health care with collaboration at the forefront. As such, cultural understanding and integration of the various agencies that come together in such a synergistic approach becomes the cornerstone of intervention.

As mentioned before, a well-recognized and substantial mental health need and treatment gap exists in LMICs. In some LMICs, this gap exceeds 90%. The gap is most severe in the area of child and adolescent mental health.[5] In attempts to reduce this gap, there is an increasing amount of research examining the effectiveness of psychological treatments (PTs) for different populations and settings. A few researchers have specifically examined the effectiveness of evidenced-based treatment (EBTs) in LMICs that have been developed in high-income countries.[5] To date, there have been several randomized controlled trials that have demonstrated promising results for common mental health problems such as depression, anxiety, and posttraumatic stress disorder. Examples include (1) interpersonal psychotherapy conducted in Uganda and India, (2) cognitive behavioral therapy (CBT) in Pakistan, and (3) cognitive processing therapy in the Democratic Republic of the Congo. Most of these studies examined adult populations, underscoring the dearth of literature in children and adolescents.[5]

However, there are 2 different viewpoints regarding the use of EBTs in LMICs. One perspective is that in order to address the treatment gap, LMICs should build and benefit from evidence in other settings (high-resource settings). Equally prevalent is the perspective that efforts should take more of an ethnographic approach and identify and test local strategies of addressing mental health problems. Addressing the substantial mental health treatment gap likely requires efforts on both fronts.[5]

What has been a common thread in the development and implementation of treatment models globally is the use of task shifting. Task shifting is the use of nonspecialists, such as primary care physicians and community health workers and lay personnel, in the delivery of care.[6–8] Language is at the heart of mental health care and is one of the prime reasons that task shifting is so important.[9] These nonspecialists usually share similar cultural backgrounds, experiences, and language of the treatment population and thus oftentimes bridge the cultural gap between specialists and the child and family in need of care. Many high-income countries have sophisticated interpreter services, but in most LMICs, these services are nonexistent. Among the 20 poorest countries in the world, 90% have more than 10 local languages and dialects and 70% of them have more than 20. To add to this linguistic diversity, documented and more commonly undocumented migration to these countries because of wars, violence, and/or economic reasons provides another layer of complexity.[9]

What is more the rule than the exception is that when a language barrier develops, the potential to engage and treat an identified child or family diminishes. Difficulties faced include the inability to translate the emotionally charged and culturally nuanced local idioms of distress into a psychiatric diagnosis, the near impossibility of discussion of confidential matters when family members act as interpreters, the inability to provide basic psychoeducation about the illness because diagnostic nomenclature equivalents are not found in the local language, and most importantly, the inability to simply communicate effectively with identified patients.[9]

Adapting evidenced-based PTs to incorporate elements that are contextually relevant and meaningful in the culture in which they are being delivered is recognized as an important step in increasing acceptability of the treatment, patient satisfaction, and ultimately, their effectiveness.[10–17] Along with language, the integration of explanatory models is one of the key elements in this adaptation process. Explanatory models have been defined as notions about an episode of sickness and its treatment that are used by all those engaged in the clinical process.[18] Thus, from the patient, family, lay counselor, local stakeholders, to specialists, understanding the cultural perspective of illness and treatment is essential. In addition, cultural adaptation attempts to maintain fidelity to the core elements of the PT, while adding certain cultural elements to enhance its acceptability and effectiveness. Chowdhary and colleagues[10] examined 8 dimensions that target cultural adaptations of PTs including language of intervention, therapist matching, cultural symbols and sayings (metaphors), cultural knowledge or content, treatment conceptualization, treatment goals, treatment methods, and consideration of treatment context. The types of PT adapted are CBT, interpersonal therapy, psychoeducation, problem-solving therapy, and dynamically oriented therapy.

Adaptations for language were frequently found to be implemented and usually went beyond the literal translation to incorporate the use of colloquial expressions to replace technical terms. Also, in some cultures, one word had several different meanings. For example, *Kokondwela* or *Kuvela-Chikondi* in Nyanja dialect in Zambia means both happiness and excitement.[5]

Therapist adaptations were also widely used. These adaptations focused on therapist-patient matching to ensure the acceptability and credibility of the therapist by emphasizing shared experiences and awareness of local customs. Some studies showed that specific training on cultural competence was implemented to enhance patient engagement. Also, cultural factors were considered in the therapist-patient relationship, for example the therapist adopting a less-directive style and the necessity to set appropriate therapeutic boundaries in others.[10]

Furthermore, with regard to therapist adaptations, the method of training a therapist is a very salient element. With the use of task shifting, it has been demonstrated that ongoing supervision and training and working collaboratively with the lay counselors throughout the treatment implementation process has been quite effective. The Apprenticeship Training Model encompasses both the trainer focusing on fidelity to the original treatment model and the lay counselor focused on any modifications needed to fit the culture and patient population.[5] Thus, the local project staff, lay counselors, and local supervisors are the primary sources and experts for the EBT adaptation.

The use of metaphors has demonstrated its significance in research literature as well. It has been shown that when metaphors are integrated into the materials of the PTs, it increased their cultural relevance. Examples included using a health calendar to monitor homework, the use of stories and local examples with characters resembling the patient's situation and background, and the use of idioms and symbols such as beads for counting thoughts and a mood ladder for rating mood.[10] Other modifications for children and adolescents in particular include traditional music to identify various emotions and different-sized sticks to scale the intensity of an emotion in multiple situations.[5]

In a study conducted by Murray and colleagues,[5] examining the effectiveness of trauma-focused cognitive behavioral therapy in children in Zambia, several cultural adaptations needed to take place. "Time out" was excluded from the treatment as a behavior modification/consequence because most families were impoverished and lived in one-room huts and thus the feasibility and effectiveness of this treatment approach was minimal. Relaxation techniques included cultural music and dance, meditation, reading a religious book, and praying. Cultural modifications of cognitive coping skills included and referenced religion to encourage positive thinking. For example, lay counselors would ask the question "What would God want you to think" in order to assist the child in constructing a more positive framework of thought.

Cultural considerations were also integrated into the content of the PT. When working with a patient with interpersonal difficulties, the therapeutic work focused on what the patient could control. Also, traditional remedies and practices were integrated into the treatment such as massage and religious therapy and additional modules such as spirituality were added to the PT manual if indicated to contextualize the treatment and address issues relevant to the cultural group.[10]

Other important adaptations included modifying the language and communication involved in explaining and discussing the mental illness in a culturally appropriate manner so that it could be well understood and reduce stigma. For instance, psychiatric labels were avoided and the problem was presented as a medical illness instead of madness. Treatment goals tended to extend beyond the depression treatment for the individual per se and focused on how the individual could be more socially accepted. Adaptations were made so that the PT could fit into the individual's broader social construct. These adaptations consisted of reducing practical barriers and improving access, for example, flexibility in scheduling, sessions delivered in a convenient setting or over the phone, and inclusion of family members.[10] PT materials were also modified so that each step in treatment did not heavily rely on literacy.

In summary, the most important and efficacious cultural adaptations when implementing EBT modalities are grounded in the dimensions of language, context, and therapist delivering the treatment. Adaptations predominantly reflected the efforts to enhance the acceptability of the PT as opposed to changing the core content of the treatment modality. With this approach, fidelity to the original PT is maintained.[10] Replacing technical terms with colloquial expressions, ensuring therapist-patient matching, and cultural competence of therapists are important considerations. Furthermore, incorporating local practices into treatment, extending the goal of treatment beyond the patient to include the family, and the simplification of treatment to include the use of nonwritten material have all been proved to be highly effective cultural adaptations for care delivery models. Thus, a high level of collaboration between specialists and nonspecialists who are native to the community and share the same cultural background and experiences is essential to the delivery of a global basic level standard of care.

Most of the literature examining cultural adaptations to treatment modalities has focused on adults. There has been very limited research looking at children and adolescents. The modest literature that does exist regarding youth and their families overall demonstrates similar effectiveness of the above-mentioned essential cultural adaptations. In addition to these, consideration should be made to address varying developmental stages and how that impacts treatment approaches. For example, working with a 7-year-old child can be quite different from working with a 16-year-old adolescent. Age in and of itself carries its own cultural contexts. Also, normally when working with children, caregivers are intricately involved. However, in some LMICs, a caregiver or supportive adult may or may not be available, and the relationship between caregiver and child may differ across cultures and contexts.[5] In some areas of sub-Saharan Africa stricken by a high prevalence of HIV/AIDS, for example, there may be a high volume of orphans. The children may be in need of mental health care, but they have lost their caregiver to illness or death. It is also important to look at family structure when working with children because extended families living within the household and multiple siblings have been shown to function either as a risk or as protective factors.[19]

Lastly, in looking at child psychopathology across cultures, it has been suggested that cultures differentially suppress (via punishment and extinction) certain child behaviors (eg, aggression) and encourage (via modeling and reinforcement) others (somatic complaints) resulting in relative levels of different types of psychopathology varying across cultures.[19] In a Vietnamese youth sample, a culture heavily influenced by Confucian tradition strongly emphasizing affective control, harmony, and self-restraint, there was a lower prevalence of externalizing problems, but at the same time, internalizing problems were more difficult to detect.[19]

Just as important in understanding cultural perspectives of illness and treatment is the understanding of cultural perspectives of wellness, resilience, self-help, and coping, as the latter intricately impacts the former. Distracting activities and strategies can be used to promote and preserve wellness. These activities may include housework, hobbies, time with family, religious/spiritual practices, support from family and friends, positive thoughts and acceptance of life's adversities, problem solving, adopting healthier lifestyles (yoga, exercise, nutrition), relaxation (music, meditation, reading books), and self-education.

Individual resilience has been described as the ability of a person to successfully adapt to or recover from stressful and traumatic experiences. Resilience is conceptualized as a multidimensional construct that incorporates personal skills and qualities together with social environments and supportive family network. Resilience is also seen as a dynamic process that changes according to cultural, developmental, and historical context of individuals, varying across gender and age. Community resilience is seen as the collective ability of a community or population to adapt and recover from adversity.[20] The rising global burden of forced migration due to armed conflict is increasingly recognized as an important issue in international public health and mental health in particular. Conflict-driven forced migration has been shown to have a strong association with higher levels of mental disorders among affected migrant populations. Although the literature is not robust, the same is true of the journey of the recent increase in undocumented minors into the United States. These journeys are wrought with separation and loss, and at times, abuse and maltreatment, placing these immigrant youth at higher risk of mental disorders. However, it has been established that many of those who experience this type of migration do not develop mental disorders despite being at risk. Individual and/or community resilience and social support have been identified as key potential mediators between forced migration experience and subsequent mental health sequelae.[20] Positive factors that influence higher resilience and positive emotional health and well-being are termed supportive and include a sense of coherence, higher family and social support, strong family and social networks, coping, religion and belief systems, individual (personal) qualities and strengths, and community support. Factors that influence lower resilience and poorer mental health include levels of acculturation; daily stressors; breakdown of family, social, and cultural networks; living conditions; gender; and continuing displaced status.[20] It is clear that the preservation and promotion of resilience especially in displaced individuals is essential to incorporate in therapeutic models and global mental health delivery systems of care. An individualized culturally informed focus when dealing with clinical encounters related to above-mentioned factors thus becomes imperative in predicting improved outcomes.

SUMMARY

There is no question that there is a significant burden of mental illness in children and families across the globe. Despite heightened awareness of the significance of global mental health and its determinants on public health, there is an increased need for innovative interventions, research, resources, and efforts devoted to this area. It has been clearly established that culture, in all of its complex dimensions and dynamics, is at the heart of this labor. In order to integrate culture into global mental health advocacy and solutions, a collaborative approach with flexibility in thinking and implementation must exist.

REFERENCES

1. Bolton P. The unknown role of mental health in global development. Yale J Biol Med 2014;87:241–9.
2. Chatterjee S, Naik S, Dubholkaar H, et al. Effectiveness of a community based intervention for people with schizophrenia and their caregivers in India (COPSI): a randomized trial. Lancet 2014;383:1385–94.
3. Patel V, Sci F, Saxena S. Transforming lives, enhancing communities – innovations in global mental health. N Engl J Med 2014;370(6):498–501.
4. Pumariega A, Rothe E, Mian A, et al. Practice parameter for cultural competence in child and adolescent psychiatric practice. J Am Acad Child Adolesc Psychiatry 2013;52:1101–15.
5. Murray L, Dorsey S, Skavenski S, et al. Identification, modification, and implementation of an evidenced based psychotherapy for children in a low-income country: the use of TF-CBT in Zambia. Int J Ment Health Syst 2013;7:24.
6. Raviola G, Eustache E, Oswald C, et al. Mental health response in Haiti in the aftermath of the 2010 earthquake: a case study for building long-term solutions. Harv Rev Psychiatry 2012;20:68–77.
7. Roberts B, Odong VN, Browne J, et al. An exploration of social determinants of health amongst internally displaced persons in northern Uganda. Confl Health 2009;3(10):1–11.
8. Sapag J, Herrera A, Trainor R, et al. Global mental health: transformative capacity building in Nicaragua. Glob Health Action 2013;6:21328.
9. Swartz L, Kilian S, Twesigye J, et al. Language, culture, and task shifting – an emerging challenge for global mental health. Glob Health Action 2014;7:23433.
10. Chowdhary N, Jotheeswaran AT, Nadkarni A, et al. The methods and outcomes of cultural adaptations of psychological treatments for depressive disorders: systematic review. Psychol Med 2014;44:1131–46.
11. Collins P, Insel T, Chockalingam A, et al. Grand challenges in global mental health: integration in research, policy and practice. PLoS Med 2013;10(4): e1001434.

12. Crumlish N, Samalani P, Sefasi A, et al. Insight, psychopathology and global functioning in schizophrenia in urban Malawi. Br J Psychiatry 2007;191:262–3.
13. Eaton J, Kakuma R, Wright A, et al. A position statement on mental health in the post-2015 development agenda. Int J Ment Health Syst 2014;8:28.
14. Fekadu A, Thornicroft G. Global mental health: perspectives from Ethiopia. Glob Health Action 2014;7:25447.
15. Maselko J, Hughes C, Cheney R. Religious social capital: its measurement and utility in the study of the social determinants of health. Soc Sci Med 2011;73(5):759–67.
16. Minas H. Global mental health and development: a thematic series. Int J Ment Health Syst 2014;8:27.
17. Minas H, Wright A, Kakuma R. Goals and organizational structure of the movement for global mental health. Int J Ment Health Syst 2014;8:31.
18. Aggarwal NK, Balaii M, Kumar S, et al. Using consumer perspectives to inform the cultural adaptation of psychological treatments for depression: a mixed methods study from South Asia. J Affect Disord 2014;163(100):88–101.
19. Weiss B, Dang M, Trung L, et al. A nationally representative epidemiological and risk factor assessment of child mental health in Vietnam. Int Perspect Psychol 2014;3(3):139–53.
20. Siriwardhana C, Ali AS, Roberts B. A systematic review of resilience and mental health outcomes of conflict-driven adult forced migrants. Confl Health 2014;8:13.

Index

Note: Page numbers of article titles are in **boldface** type.

Child Adolesc Psychiatric Clin N Am 24 (2015) 831–840
http://dx.doi.org/10.1016/S1056-4993(15)00071-1 **childpsych.theclinics.com**

G

H

I

N

O

P

S

T

U

V

United States Postal Service

Statement of Ownership, Management, and Circulation (All Periodicals Publications Except Requestor Publications)

1. Publication Title Child and Adolescent Psychiatric Clinics of North America	2. Publication Number 0 1 1 - 3 6 8	3. Filing Date 9/18/15
4. Issue Frequency Jan, Apr, Jul, Oct	5. Number of Issues Published Annually 4	6. Annual Subscription Price $310.00
7. Complete Mailing Address of Known Office of Publication (*Not printer*) (*Street, city, county, state, and ZIP+4®*) Elsevier Inc. 360 Park Avenue South New York, NY 10010-1710		Contact Person Stephen R. Bushing Telephone (Include area code) 215-239-3688

8. Complete Mailing Address of Headquarters or General Business Office of Publisher (*Not printer*)

Elsevier Inc., 360 Park Avenue South, New York, NY 10010-1710

9. Full Names and Complete Mailing Addresses of Publisher, Editor, and Managing Editor (*Do not leave blank*)

Publisher (*Name and complete mailing address*)

Linda Belfus, Elsevier Inc., 1600 John F. Kennedy Blvd., Suite 1800, Philadelphia, PA 19103

Editor (*Name and complete mailing address*)

Lauren Boyle, Elsevier Inc., 1600 John F. Kennedy Blvd., Suite 1800, Philadelphia, PA 19103-2899

Managing Editor (*Name and complete mailing address*)

Adrianne Brigido, Elsevier Inc., 1600 John F. Kennedy Blvd., Suite 1800, Philadelphia, PA 19103-2899

10. Owner (*Do not leave blank. If the publication is owned by a corporation, give the name and address of the corporation immediately followed by the names and addresses of all stockholders owning or holding 1 percent or more of the total amount of stock. If not owned by a corporation, give the names and addresses of the individual owners. If owned by a partnership or other unincorporated firm, give its name and address as well as those of each individual owner. If the publication is published by a nonprofit organization, give its name and address.*)

Full Name	Complete Mailing Address
Wholly owned subsidiary of	1600 John F. Kennedy Blvd, Ste. 1800
Reed/Elsevier, US holdings	Philadelphia, PA 19103-2899

11. Known Bondholders, Mortgagees, and Other Security Holders Owning or Holding 1 Percent or More of Total Amount of Bonds, Mortgages, or Other Securities. If none, check box → ☐ None

Full Name	Complete Mailing Address
N/A	

12. Tax Status (*For completion by nonprofit organizations authorized to mail at nonprofit rates*) (*Check one*)
The purpose, function, and nonprofit status of this organization and the exempt status for federal income tax purposes:
☐ Has Not Changed During Preceding 12 Months
☐ Has Changed During Preceding 12 Months (*Publisher must submit explanation of change with this statement*)

13. Publication Title Child and Adolescent Psychiatric Clinics of North America	14. Issue Date for Circulation Data Below July 2015

PS Form 3526, July 2014 (Page 1 of 3 (Instructions Page 3)) PSN 7530-01-000-9931 **PRIVACY NOTICE**: See our Privacy policy in www.usps.com

15. Extent and Nature of Circulation			Average No. Copies Each Issue During Preceding 12 Months	No. Copies of Single Issue Published Nearest to Filing Date
a. Total Number of Copies (*Net press run*)			470	396
b. Legitimate Paid and Or Requested Distribution (By Mail and Outside the Mail)	(1)	Mailed Outside County Paid/Requested Mail Subscriptions stated on PS Form 3541. (*Include paid distribution above nominal rate, advertiser's proof copies and exchange copies*)	229	192
	(2)	Mailed In-County Paid/Requested Mail Subscriptions stated on PS Form 3541. (*Include paid distribution above nominal rate, advertiser's proof copies and exchange copies*)		
	(3)	Paid Distribution Outside the Mails Including Sales Through Dealers And Carriers, Street Vendors, Counter Sales, and Other Paid Distribution Outside USPS®	67	66
	(4)	Paid Distribution by Other Classes of Mail Through the USPS (e.g. First-Class Mail®)		
c. Total Paid and or Requested Circulation (*Sum of 15b (1), (2), (3), and (4)*) ►			296	258
d. Free or Nominal Rate Distribution (By Mail and Outside the Mail)	(1)	Free or Nominal Rate Outside-County Copies included on PS Form 3541	74	75
	(2)	Free or Nominal Rate in-County Copies included on PS Form 3541		
	(3)	Free or Nominal Rate Copies mailed at Other classes Through the USPS (e.g. First-Class Mail®)		
	(4)	Free or Nominal Rate Distribution Outside the Mail (*Carriers or Other means*)		
e. Total Nonrequested Distribution (Sum of 15d (1), (2), (3) and (4)			74	75
f. Total Distribution (Sum of 15c and 15e) ►			370	333
g. Copies not Distributed (See instructions to publishers #4 (page #3)) ►			100	63
h. Total (Sum of 15f and g)			470	396
i. Percent Paid and/or Requested Circulation (15c divided by 15f times 100) ►			80.00%	77.48%

* If you are claiming electronic copies go to line 16 on page 3. If you are not claiming Electronic copies, skip to line 17 on page 3

16. Electronic Copy Circulation	*Average No. Copies Each Issue During Preceding 12 Months*	*No. Copies of Single Issue Published Nearest to Filing Date*
a. Paid Electronic Copies		
b. Total paid Print Copies (Line 15c) + Paid Electronic copies (Line 16a)		
c. Total Print Distribution (Line 15f) + Paid Electronic Copies (Line 16a)		
d. Percent Paid (Both Print & Electronic copies) (16b divided by 16c X 100)		
I certify that 50% of all my distributed copies (electronic and print) are paid above a nominal price		

17. Publication of Statement of Ownership
If the publication is a general publication, publication of this statement is required. Will be printed in the *__October 2015__* *issue of this publication.*

18. Signature and Title of Editor, Publisher, Business Manager, or Owner	Date
Stephen R. Bushing Stephen R. Bushing – Inventory Distribution Coordinator	September 18, 2015

I certify that all information furnished on this form is true and complete. I understand that anyone who furnishes false or misleading information on this form or who omits material or information requested on the form may be subject to criminal sanctions (including fines and imprisonment) and/or civil sanctions (including civil penalties).

PS Form 3526, July 2014 (Page 3 of 3)

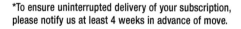

Printed and bound by CPI Group (UK) Ltd, Croydon, CR0 4YY
07/10/2024
01040498-0018